THE BURDEN OF SYMPATHY

THE BURDEN OF SYMPATHY

How Families Cope with Mental Illness

DAVID A. KARP

OXFORD
UNIVERSITY PRESS

2001

OXFORD
UNIVERSITY PRESS

Oxford New York

Athens Auckland Bangkok Bogotá Buenos Aires
Calcutta Cape Town Dar es Salaam Delhi Florence
Hong Kong Istanbul Karachi Kuala Lumpur
Madrid Melbourne Mexico City Mumbai
Nairobi Paris São Paulo Singapore Taipei
Tokyo Toronto Warsaw

and associated companies in
Berlin Ibadan

Copyright © 2001 Oxford University Press, Inc.

Published by Oxford University Press, Inc.
198 Madison Avenue, New York, New York 10016

Oxford is a registered trademark of Oxford University Press

LIBRARY OF CONGRESS CATALOGING-IN-PUBLICATION DATA
Karp, David Allen, 1944–
The Burden of sympathy : how families cope with mental illness / by David A. Karp.
p. cm. Includes bibliographical references and index.
ISBN 0-19-512315-8
1. Mentally ill—Home care. 2. Mentally ill—Family relationships.
3. Caregivers. I. Title

RC439.5.K37 2001 362.2'0422—dc21 99-058513

135798642
Printed in the United States of America
on acid-free paper

*For all the Family and Friends at MDDA
and especially for Tom Schaeffer,
who believed that "out of all the apparently
evil, dark, and painful stuff,
our job is to make flowers grow."*

CONTENTS

ACKNOWLEDGMENTS

The Burden of Sympathy tells the second half of a story I began in a previous book, *Speaking of Sadness*. Because *Speaking of Sadness* emerged so significantly from my own difficulties with depression, I had a visceral sense for the validity of my arguments as I did the writing. This book depended more on "distance learning" since I have not had firsthand experience caring for a mentally ill family member. That being so, the completion of this enterprise required substantial reliance on colleagues, friends, and family caregivers who helped to shape my ideas or to provide an insider's perspective on the adequacy of my analyses.

I consider myself unusually fortunate that among my closest friends are two colleagues at Boston College. My ongoing conversations with Charlie Derber and John Williamson are always enormously engaging. Their wisdom and compassion help me to live life more gracefully. They are also extraordinarily gifted social scientists whose advice invariably makes my work better. I am deeply appreciative that Charlie and John are always willing to let me share the moments of doubt, confusion, and pleasure that all writers experience.

Another longtime friend, Bill Yoels, has been my collaborator on several books and articles since we first met in 1971. He has read every word I have written for nearly three decades. Nothing I write goes off to a professional journal or book publisher until it gets Bill's approval. I admire his sociological imagination, his playfulness with ideas, his ironic wit, his intellectual integrity, and his honesty about the things I write. Bill has also been a great friend when my needs went far beyond sociological counsel.

The relationships that can come of it are among the most gratifying payoffs of doing ethnographic research. When I began this project I asked the members of a "Family and Friends" support group at McLean's hospital in Belmont, Massachusetts, whether I might join them, strictly as an observer. They have been exceedingly gracious in supporting this work from the outset. I continue to sit in on the group nearly every Wednesday night because I continue to learn new things. I also go because I now count several group members among my friends. Finally, I go because, in simple human terms, I want to hear how their always difficult, poignant, and courageous stories continue to unfold. You will see just how significantly my thinking about caregiving has been influenced by what I see, hear, and feel in that group.

About a year ago, the MDDA (The Manic Depressive and Depressive Association) Chapter at McLean's changed its rules. I never learned what precipitated the change, but the guidelines read in each of the "sharing and caring" groups at the start of meetings now explicitly deny access to "observers." When I first heard the new rule and volunteered to leave, Jim, one of the group's mainstays told me, "Oh no, we've discussed it and that rule doesn't apply to you. We want you to stay. You've been here for a long time and, besides, you're going to tell our side of the story." The communication both pleased and concerned me. The vote of confidence was terrific. However, being seen as a spokesperson of sorts made my task feel far more weighty. I hope that Jim and every other person I've met in the support group would approve of what I have written.

Several students, colleagues, and caregivers read drafts of this book as I went along. Sometimes they advised me about theoretical directions. Sometimes they sensitized me to errors, misplaced emphases, or important omissions. Let me thank Michele Carpentieri, Marjorie DeVault, Elizabeth Doherty, Barry Feldman, Arthur Frank, Sigrid Johnson, Christina Johnson-Levetin, Aimee Marlow, Nancy Redding, Alice Schaeffer, Tom Schaeffer, Nancy Sharby, Valaya Tanarugsachock, and Diane Watts-Roy. I hope I have done justice to your insights. There are others whom I cannot acknowledge by name. Their wish for confidentiality is understandable. Unfortunately, it reflects America's continuing and disheartening ignorance about mental illness. Thank you all.

As I approach my thirtieth year teaching at Boston College I once again feel lucky to have spent my working life at such a humane and supportive institution. A Boston College Research Incentive Grant helped to get this work off the ground. Later, a Research Expense Grant from the university kept the momentum going. I am also grateful to the American Sociological Association for awarding me a grant as part of a "Fund for the Advancement of the Discipline." These sources of financial aid freed me from some of the more onerous tasks associated with in-depth interview research and maximized the time I could spend reading, thinking about the data, and writing.

Of course, my work depends completely on the real "experts." I feel tremendously privileged to have heard the accounts of the sixty people whose words constitute the core of this effort. They were remarkably candid with me about a very painful aspect of their lives. Each person is a reminder that maintaining commitments when they are most sorely tested is an act of great courage and heroism. If it is ever demanded of me, I hope I can honor my obligations as well as the people who speak throughout this book. I have tried to illuminate the commonalties they faced in caring for someone they love with a mental illness. Although it does not diminish the tragedy of catastrophic illness, my most profound hope is that by recognizing themselves in the accounts of others, caregivers who read this book will feel less alone in their struggle.

Shortly after she completed two years of Peace Corps service in Western Africa, I took advantage of my daughter Alyssa's temporary unemployment by having her proofread the manuscript. It was also fun to have her as a travel companion when I gave occasional talks on my research. While my son, Peter, kids me about all the time I spend at home, I think he understands that what I do actually qualifies as "work." Finally, as always, I am deeply indebted to my wife, Darleen. I simply could not do my writing without her support, encouragement, love, and care.

D.A.K
Chestnut Hill
January 2001

THE BURDEN OF SYMPATHY

ONE

Illness and Obligation

As little as we know of illness, we know even less of
care. As much as the ill person's experience is denied,
the caregiver's experience is denied more completely.

ARTHUR FRANK, *At the Will of the Body*

The sequence of events beginning nearly four years ago in Leslie's
life was not unlike the plot in a Steven King novel. At first, the
incidences seemed pretty insignificant, although each did cause momentary wonder and worry. After a slightly unsettling event, life
returns to its normal, relatively uncomplicated rhythm. At a point,
though, the disturbing events become more frequent and seem to
constitute a pattern. Characters may now begin to confide uneasy
feelings to each other about what has been happening, while finding
ways to deny that anything is badly amiss. At a point, the scary
problems become so intrusive that the now badly frightened characters know something must be terribly wrong, although they still
can't comprehend what is going on. They begin an earnest search
for answers, but the underlying cause of the expanding strangeness
eludes them. Finally, such awful events occur that life becomes a
frantic effort to solve, escape, or somehow eradicate the clear horror
that now dominates every waking moment, even haunting their
dreams.

Because of the sheer complexity of her son's illness and her need
to talk about it, Leslie and I spoke on three separate occasions.
Near the beginning of our first conversation she said that "so much

has happened in three years that I don't even know where to begin. ... It's overwhelming." There was, though, one thing that she absolutely wanted to bring up right away and have me understand. Through a phone conversation prior to our meeting, Leslie knew that I was interested in the "boundaries of obligation." Before I could ask my first question she told me that "my boundaries are very different from other people's." She went on to explain that "Mike has the potential for violence. And ... because I know this is being recorded, it's really important to me for you to know that he is innately a very, very sweet and kind person. But [because of] his disease he gets very paranoid. His disease has made him a danger to others. ... I mean, he wouldn't even step on a bug, you know? But this illness is so [awful] and he has attacked his brother, attacked his sister." Throughout our nearly ten hours of talk, Leslie repeatedly sought assurance that I would not confuse Mike with his disease.

The first hints of a problem began when Mike was in the sixth grade. Unlike most ten-year-old boys, "he hated sports. He just loved to read and so I just figured, 'Well, most boys are out there playing ball or whatever, and Mike doesn't want to do that. He reads. His life is books. So he was different in that way.' " Because Mike also wore glasses and was skinny "he didn't really fit in. ... He used to be teased a lot." Later in high school, "kids used to put tacks on his chair ... [and] one kid on the school bus held a bottle of shampoo over his head and ... it came down all over him and ... the bus driver never did anything." Such mistreatment would be unsettling for any parent, but more ominous was a call from Mike's sixth grade teacher who felt obliged to tell Leslie that "Mike looks at me like he wants to kill me." Since Mike was "a very kind child and. ... an excellent student [and] was a good kid at home, I thought the teacher was crazy." Three years later the family had moved to the Midwest, Mike's grades began a dramatic plunge, and his new ninth grade teacher reported in a conference, "Gee, he looks at me like he wants to kill me." This was the beginning of "a crescendoing ... an escalation of signs of trouble."

By the ninth grade it was plain that Mike was significantly distressed. "He started to get very poor grades. . . . He would sit in the back of the class and read his own books . . . books like history [and] philosophy." By the time he was a senior Mike had "become very difficult" and, Leslie recalled, "I would call his guidance counselor in high school—the poor man—[and] I would start crying on the phone. . . . But everyone would say, 'Oh, Mike's okay. He'll be all right.' " As much as they wanted to believe that Mike was all right, Leslie and her husband Bob now openly spoke about getting him counseling and even contemplated finding a private high school where he might fit in more easily. The belief that Mike's behavior reflected normal adolescent confusion became somewhat more untenable after a particular incident. Along with some friends, Mike pulled a prank that was very unsettling to a neighbor. Because Mike had been driving the family car and someone noted the license number, the police arrived at their home. Leslie promised to call the other boys' parents, and with that the police left. She then described to me the scene as she later tried to talk with her son:

> I said, "Mike, don't you understand that . . . it was funny to you
> kids, but to this man [it's not funny]." And Mike, well, he couldn't
> see it. And so, I just put my hands on his shoulders, and I put them
> gently, and I said, "I just want you to understand what it meant to
> this man." And all of a sudden, he like pushed me away. We were
> in the kitchen, and there was a basket of fruit—grapefruit, oranges.
> And he picked them up, one by one, and hurled them against the
> wall. I mean, so that there was, you know, pulp and juice. I mean
> the kitchen, the family room, there was this splattered fruit every-
> where. And I was, like, numb. I just said, "What are you doing?"
> But I was just like, frozen. And then he said, "I have to take a walk."
> Well, by now it was like midnight; it was pitch black. He walked out
> of the house. I didn't know what to do. I didn't know whether to
> call the police. You know, I thought, "Well, I'll wait. He'll come
> back." Well, I found my daughter, she's two and a half years younger

than he is. This had woken her up. She was sitting on the stairs, crying, saying, you know, "Why does he do things like this?" So, I talked to her and hugged her. She went back for a while to bed. And I started scrubbing this pulp and this juice and this mess that was all over. And I'm . . . meticulous at housekeeping. . . . So I spent the entire night, from like 1:00 A.M. to 6:00 A.M. scrubbing this mess, and he never came home.

Just as they would respond so many times before eventually accepting Mike's diagnosis of "schizo-affective disorder," Leslie and Bob hoped that one change or another would solve the problem. Despite his low grades in high school, Mike achieved an exceedingly high score on the SAT tests and was admitted to a local college with a scholarship. She told me that "we both just really hoped that he would go to college and would find his niche there, and that would solve everything." They were, therefore, chagrined when Mike's first semester grades were so poor that he lost his scholarship. Nevertheless, despite heavy drinking and probable drug use, Mike continued to get by. Things seemed to change for the better when he took a course in Russian language and excelled. He changed his major to Russian Language and Literature, was admitted into a junior year abroad program, and, most important, told his parents, "I finally found somewhere where I fit in." Leslie remembered, "I [was] feeling euphoric. Oh, he's happy and everything's going to be fine."

Aside from hoping that a newfound love for language and foreign culture would turn things around, Leslie admitted with some embarrassment that she was happy to have her son leave for a year. She said, "Well, I'm really ashamed of this. The thought of him being inaccessible for twelve months was a wonderful thought to me. I was actually delighted that he was accepted because, God forgive me, I knew that I wouldn't set eyes on him again for twelve months, that he'd be too far away." She went on to explain, "See, he [still] didn't have any kind of diagnosis. I just thought I loved him but I couldn't stand him." Not only did they get a respite from their son's difficult behaviors, they also began to feel more hopeful that Mike's "adolescent rebellion" was over. "He got A's in his classes and 'he sounded good,' so we did think, 'Eureka!' you know?" Such optimism was, however, short-lived.

Things began to unravel completely after an "accident." As they later pieced it together, Mike had, in fact, purposely set his dorm room desk on fire. Although school officials accepted his account, Mike began to lose interest in his classes, "traveled around Russia for the next half a year, got no credit . . . and [finally] came home. . . . He looked terrible. He's very tall and must have weighed 120 pounds. I mean he was a walking skeleton. . . . God forgive us, we couldn't stand him. He was slovenly. . . . He wasn't shaving. He wasn't bathing." Leslie now understands all of these as "signs of mental illness," but at that moment could not recognize his behavior for what it was. She was, though, "thinking something is seriously wrong here." Despite their grave misgivings, Mike insisted that it would be best for him to spend time with friends on the West Coast, and Leslie reluctantly paid for the plane ticket. A short time later, he was home again, having alienated friends, lost multiple jobs, and squandered the money urgently and repeatedly wired to him via Western Union. By now, Leslie could not dismiss mental illness as an explanation for the years of turmoil, which began so subtly in the sixth grade. Our conversation proceeded this way:

This is absorbing your life at this point?

Oh, my God. Oh, yes. I knew he was ill. And there was something on the news about one of these incidents where a postal clerk . . . a disgruntled person, had gone in and shot other people. And in my heart, I felt that my son could do, and might do, something like this. I just had the feeling in my heart that my son was capable of killing, because I was sure at this point . . . that he was crazy, and that he was capable of killing. And I said to my husband, we were watching the news, and this thing was on the news, and I said, "You know, I think Mike is capable of that." And he said, "What??!!" He

said, "You're crazy." I said, "Don't you feel that he is capable of
hurting someone?" He said, "No!"

So did that make you feel that you were off the beam?

I felt in my heart that I wasn't off the beam. . . . So, finally, once
again he called and needed money, and we just said, "Forget it," you
know? "The only money you'll get from us is a plane ticket back
here. You have to come home." And we weren't going to give him
money to buy it. We said, "We'll get the plane ticket. You go to the
airport, and the ticket will be there."

*So by this time you really had to start taking precautions about how
you sent money.*

Oh, yes, yeah. . . . So he came back, and I picked him up at the
airport that day. . . . Anyway, so he came home, and we have a finished basement, and I had turned his room upstairs into a guest
room, with his knowledge. . . . So, for the first couple of weeks, we
just never saw him. He just slept, slept, slept. At first I thought,
"Well, sure, he's tired." Then I began to think, "He's depressed. He's
always in bed." And I tried to talk to him about it. The other thing
. . . well, we kept finding, like broken glass and stuff. And I thought,
"Well, he's clumsy. He's breaking stuff. He's dropping things." And
I was finding, like, marks on the walls and on the floors. It turns
out, he was spitting. He was spitting all over the walls and the floor,
but I didn't realize that. I mean, you don't expect that your kid is
spitting everywhere. So, we would find broken glass, and all I said
was, "Mike, if you break a glass by accident, make sure you clean it
up, so no one gets cut." So, one day I went down to his room—he
did his own laundry, but he had left it upstairs, and I wanted to
stick it in his room, and get it out of the way. And I walked into
his room, and his dresser is carved up. Huge letters. There were
three drawers. On each drawer was a huge word—FUCK . . . THIS . . .
SHIT. He had to have spent the whole night [doing it]. Plus, there

were holes bored into it. There was no more denying it. . . . This kid
was really sick.

As she continued to detail her son's increasingly strange, destructive, and threatening behaviors, Leslie tried to convey just how incredibly awful she found the unfolding of her son's illness. At various points she said: "Sometimes I think it would be easier if he
had cancer. His disease is so dreadful." "When all this hell, this
sheer hell broke loose . . . we were in such agony." "Not to sound
melodramatic, but it's worse than a movie. I mean, I can't believe
it's my life, my son's life." "We don't have a life. We don't have a
life." "I just look at him and my heart breaks all the time." "It's
always on my mind. It's my existence. I am obsessed with my son's
illness. His illness is my life." As her account moved from one
horrible scene to another, several involving physical violence, the
profundity of Leslie's pain became more palpable. By now, also, her
two younger children (a seventeen-year-old daughter and fourteen-
year-old son) had become thoroughly traumatized. Her daughter,
for example, "was barricading her door at night, piling stuff up
against it, and hung bells on her door so that if the door moved
the bells would jingle." Their son was "using one of those bars
advertised on TV. . . . He was locking himself in with that at night."

By the time of our interview, Mike had already been hospitalized
five times. Each hospitalization was preceded by extreme psychosis
and overtly threatening behavior. Perhaps, though, it was the first
hospitalization that was the most agonizing for Leslie and her family. The episode leading up to the hospitalization began on a Thurs-
day evening. Mike was breaking things and throwing them in a
dumpster. By the time he was done, "he had broken over $2000
worth of stuff. . . . He would take the pool cue—there were recessed
lights in the ceiling—and he was breaking all of those. He started
breaking things and he didn't care if we knew." After an emergency
consultation with a psychologist, Leslie and Bob were told that Mike
should be hospitalized immediately. At first, they said, "No." "Even
though we knew it was serious, we thought she [the psychologist]

just went off the deep end. [We thought], 'All he needs is some counseling.' " They returned home, hoping to handle things themselves, but the next day brought an even more frightening event.

After failing to register, as planned, at a local college, "Mike walked into the house, picked up a kitchen chair and slammed it on the floor, breaking the chair and putting a hole in the floor." His younger brother, unable to contain himself, screamed, "I am sick of this." Mike then "grabbed Josh and brought his knee into Josh's stomach, and he was holding him there, and he said, 'Which way do you want to bleed to death?'" Following an hysterical call from Josh, Leslie rushed home and, after being threatened herself, fled to a neighbor's home to call a crisis team. On her way she spotted a police car and flagged it down. The police escorted her home and although Mike was still talking strangely, "He didn't look crazy. He looks like he's fine, you know? And I had cleaned up everything he had broken. There was no evidence of the stuff he had been smashing." After a brief talk, the police left. Later, Leslie would say, "I just couldn't believe the police were there and I sent them away." By the time her husband returned home, it was plain that Mike had to be removed from the house. The whole family spent a harrowing weekend until Bob could get to a local district court on Monday. Here is how their son was removed from his own home:

> So, the courthouse opened at 9:00, and my husband was down there at 9:00. And I'm thinking to myself, "Oh, this will have to take a few hours, at least." I just didn't want it to happen. So, I'm thinking, "He'll be there for hours. We've got at least a few hours." He was back within half an hour, and he said, "They'll be here in a few minutes." And sure enough, within ten minutes [they arrived]. . . . Now, no one prepared us, no one prepared us for the horror that this would be. They sent two police cars. Josh was in school. Andrea was home, because it was semester break. Two police cars. Mike was asleep. They sent in four officers. They went downstairs to his room, burst in on him, grabbed him and put handcuffs on him, while he's

barely awake, and like, even if you're in your right frame of mind you'd be confused. And so, here is this very sick person. And he is going, "This is a mistake. This is a mistake." He said, "Just ask my dad." My husband was so distraught. This was probably the worst day of our lives. My husband was so distraught. He was trying not to sob. Andrea was hysterical. She was hysterical. So, I'm holding Andrea. And the cops are taking Mike. I don't think he even had shoes on. It was January. He couldn't get a coat on, because he was handcuffed, you know, behind his back. I forget. . . . I think Mike's saying something like, "Could I please put my shoes on?" I . . . threw a jacket over his shoulders, maybe. And they took him away. And my husband is sobbing, Andrea's sobbing, I'm sobbing, we are just all sobbing.

And so, they took him to the [names town] District Court, and they put him in a jail cell. And, after a while we composed ourselves, and we went down to the courthouse. And he had to go before the judge. And they asked us if we wanted to go into the courtroom. And I couldn't. I mean, he was given a public defender. . . . This was taking hours now. And they interviewed us, and then had to go talk to Mike. And all of this was taking forever, taking forever. And then, finally, after all of that, he told us that he would recommend that Mike be hospitalized. . . . So, he had to go to [names a health center], which is a state hospital, an acute care facility. But they put him back in the jail cell. He sat in a jail cell from 9:30 in the morning until 6:00 at night, just sitting in a jail cell. And he was mentally ill. It doesn't seem right, the whole thing. We were never prepared for four police officers putting him in handcuffs. I mean, this person, he's sick. It was a nightmare. It was just a nightmare.

The circumstances I have described certainly suggest the degree to which Mike's illness has become a nightmare for a whole family. Since I have not spoken with Leslie's husband or children I cannot know just how completely mental illness has enveloped each of them. From her account, though, I believe that Leslie, like all the mothers with whom I have spoken, has found it more difficult than

other family members to distance herself from a child's catastrophic
illness. She told me, "I honestly don't think there is a minute of
the day that I am not thinking about . . . my son. I wake up thinking
about him. I go to bed thinking about him. If I wake up in the
middle of the night . . . I think of him. . . . It's my existence. He's
my child." Leslie repeatedly worried aloud about the ways her "ob-
session" with Mike's illness might be injuring her husband and
children. Several times, she expressed concern that "I am failing
my other children and failing my husband" because "I am stuck
in this little world of my son and me."

The parts of our conversation about the division of the caregiving labor in Leslie's family were instructive. During his lengthy hospitalizations, Leslie visited her son nearly every day, but did not
expect anything approaching such an involvement from her children. Josh is "away at school and he really can't get back here."
"Andrea," she explained, "is very sympathetic. I mean, she loves
him, but she finds it very difficult to go there [the hospital] and
visit him. So, she's gone a few times, but she doesn't go and I
understand. She just finds it too hard. She needs that space." When
our conversation turned to her relationship with Bob, she was willing to say, "If I were my husband, I'd want to leave me at this
point." At the same time, she also expressed frustration that Bob
did not understand her feelings as a mother. Leslie spoke for most
of the mothers in this study when she lamented that her husband
"puts things in compartments. He can go to work and he puts it
out of his mind. But with me . . . it colors everything I do and he
doesn't understand this." She went on to say:

> He's my child. I gave birth to him. I had this intense bonding with
> him when he was born, and he was just . . . you know, so perfect and
> beautiful. . . . And I mean, I still love him. You know, he's my child.
> He's part of my body. And my husband, I try to explain that to him,
> and he doesn't quite get it. . . . I just remember holding him as an
> infant, and it would feel like we were one, you know? I'd have him
> in my arms and I just felt like we were one. And I don't know
> whether it was because he was . . . my first child, or what I really

hoped for him. What I hoped for all of my children [was] for them just to be happy, because as a child I had a wonderful mother, a wonderful mother, but I was afraid a lot. I was unhappy a lot. And I just did not want that for my children.

Aside from the particular bond that arises from giving birth, Leslie felt that her special affinity with Mike comes from her own troubled childhood. While Bob grew up in a *"Leave it to Beaver...* adorable little white house in the country [and] never heard his parents argue... I believe that my father was mentally ill. My father did dreadful things [and] I was afraid of him." As a result, Leslie believes she feels Mike's pain in a way that Bob cannot. She told me that "this illness, this pain that he's in, it's unbearable to me. His pain is my pain.... My husband doesn't see it like that and finds it hard to understand how I can feel it so intensely.... I think he gets my son's pain [but] he doesn't internalize it the way I do." Leslie's inability to distance herself from the caretaking role has created difficulties in her marriage.

> It's been really hard on my relationship with my husband.... At the beginning it drew us closer, that horrendous time when we had to get the court order, and they dragged him out of the house in handcuffs. We were just so close, we just held each other, and he cried and I cried, and we said, you know, "We have to hold on to each other." And we were so close. But now, it's sort of a wedge, because... it's much easier for him to separate it. You know, he goes to work; he can put Mike out of his mind when he goes. Thank God he can do that. I mean, he's under a lot of stress at work. But I can't seem to ever do that.... I've tried to explain it to him. It's part of me; he's my child. I feel like I just can't divorce myself from it. And I know my husband takes it personally.... I've let it come between us.

Mental illness is a contagious disease in its effects on others. After three years it had dangerously raised the temperature of Leslie's marriage and she is afraid that her relative neglect of Andrea and Josh could spawn permanent resentment. In describing the spread of the disease, Leslie noted that Andrea's "serious relationship" with a boyfriend ended because "[He] just can't handle what's going on with [our] family." Further, because she worries about the genetic inheritability of schizophrenia, Leslie "truly hope[s] that Mike never has children." She also said, "I always used to think . . . I'd love to be a grandparent, but now I'm thinking 'I'm not sure I want to have grandchildren. I'm not sure that Josh and Andrea should have children,' [although] I would never tell them that."

The transmissibility of mental illness is, however, most obvious in its impact on Leslie herself. She admitted to me with some hesitation that her own depression had grown to the point where [she] "actually felt suicidal." Although she has suffered from periods of depression in the past, Leslie understands that her current debilitating insomnia is intimately connected with Mike's plight. When I asked about her capacity to distance herself from Mike's illness, she told me, "Oh, I have a very long way to go, a very long way. . . . [Right now] I feel like I will drown . . . if I don't get a little more [distant]. . . . [But] I'm his mother. It's very, very difficult for me not to be there." Intellectually, Leslie may understand the wisdom of gaining distance from her son's problems. However, the prescription to withdraw from a child's trouble is emotionally counterintuitive. Leslie cannot easily accept that profound empathy for her child's pain might be an obstacle to greater wellness. Numerous interviews affirm that it is an exceedingly hard lesson for *any* mother to learn.

⤶

Over a three-year period I listened to many parents like Leslie talk about the heartache associated with a child's mental illness. I have also interviewed children of emotionally sick parents, spouses with a mentally ill partner, and siblings of those suffering from depression, manic-depression, or schizophrenia. As with Leslie, each has a unique story to tell about what it is like to care for a sick family member. Every relationship poses distinctive challenges as individuals struggle to understand the pain of another's illness and its consequences. At the same time, my lengthy conversations with the family members of people with a major mental illness reveal strong regularities. Caregivers must negotiate the boundaries of their involvement with the sick, and, in their efforts to do this, there are striking similarities that transcend the particularities of each circumstance.[1] My central purpose in this book is to illuminate these commonalties. I am most primarily interested in how family members construct obligations to someone with a serious emotional illness and then deal with the inevitable difficulties in honoring their commitment.

A book's integrity requires that its author approach a fundamental question or problem that provides a consolidating theme from beginning to end. Substantively, this book is about the social tango between emotionally ill people and those who try to help them. In an even more encompassing way, the difficult task of caring for a sick person provides a conceptual space for examining the essential nature of people's obligations and responsibilities to each other. Nearly every general theory concerned with understanding social order assumes that expectations of reciprocity and exchange constitute the essential foundation of organized society. "Obligation," the theorist Georg Simmel wrote, "belongs among those 'microscopic,' but infinitely tough threads which tie one element of society to another, and thus eventually all of them together in a stable collective life."[2] In this way, the relationship between sick people and their caregivers exposes the limits of obligation, responsibility, empathy, understanding, and sympathy in *all* relationships. This study of family caregivers, therefore, speaks to no less a question than "What do we owe each other?"[3]

The relationship between sick people and those close to them may be the quintessential case for thinking about the moral and social foundations of all human relationships. Severe illness, because it so thoroughly disrupts family life, calls attention to the taken-for-granted, normally invisible boundaries of social relationships. Prolonged illness makes demands on a child, parent, spouse, or sibling that test the relative strength of the ties that bind us together. In a beautifully written book, based on her experience with "chronic fatigue syndrome," Kat Duff wisely advises that "Not only is it better for the sick to be left alone at times, it is also better for the well to leave them at times. Healthy people can be contaminated by the gloom and depression of the ailing if they come too close or have too much sympathy."[4] The accounts in this book will show that sustaining an appropriate level of involvement with a mentally ill child, parent, sibling, or spouse is extraordinarily difficult.

Shortly into this project, interviews of the sort I did with Leslie made me realize that an exclusive focus on the purely social mandates of duty, responsibility, and obligation would be incomplete. The sixty conversations forming the core of this book affirmed the extraordinary power of love in sustaining ties with a mentally ill family member.[5] Even when an ill person treated them with anger and disdain, denied that they were sick, completely disrupted the coherence of everyday life, and did things that were incomprehensible, distressing beyond measure, socially repugnant, or downright dangerous, love often kept caregivers caring. Throughout this book, therefore, one of my tasks will be to show how responsibility, obligation, duty, *and* love mix in different combinations to sustain family ties. Later chapters illuminate how the chemistry of moral requirements and heartfelt emotions may be different for men and women and different for parents, spouses, children, and siblings of mentally ill people.[6] You will see how the ongoing construction of caregiving boundaries reflects the shifting combinations of reason and emotion, of head and heart, that connect kin over the evolving history of a person's mental illness.

The novelist Umberto Eco has written that "a writer is what a book uses to make a second book." In fact, the questions I am raising about our capacity to care have evolved over several years and are intimately linked to an earlier book I wrote on depression. *Speaking of Sadness* arose from my own more than twenty-year history with depression.[7] Based on my experience and fifty lengthy conversations with persons who have been diagnosed and treated for clinical depression, I wanted most primarily to understand how those afflicted make sense of their illness. My agenda centered less on matters of cause and cure than on the way depressed people impose order, coherence, and meaning onto a life situation that seems so utterly incoherent, problematic, and, literally, meaningless. I tried to describe what depression "feels like" and how those feelings must be interpreted within a social context.

One of my colleagues at Boston College once described writing as like dropping a feather down a well and waiting to hear something. So, I was delighted when *Speaking of Sadness* was applauded in a *New York Times Book Review* article and have been grateful for the several opportunities to talk about my work with community groups, academic audiences, and the media.[8] Most gratifying, though, has been the steady stream of communications from readers who tell me that my book has somehow been important to them. It is exhilarating to learn that I have well enough captured the phenomenology of depression so that readers see themselves in the data and understand their experiences differently because of my analysis.

Nearly always the letters, e-mail messages, and occasional phone calls thank me for writing the book and then launch into a description of the writer's own experience with mental illness. Among these communications, though, have been several from people who are trying their best to help someone they care about who has been flattened by depression. In one case, I began an e-mail correspondence with a man in the Midwest, and when I casually offered the opinion that a book on the experiences of family caregivers might be worthwhile, he responded:

> Please, undertake such a project!! You are correct in surmising that there are a variety of stories about the "careers" of those who have a depressed person in the family. . . . Your descriptions of depression, depressed people and the stages of their illness were so accurate that I thought you must have been living with Linda and myself. In our

case, the combination of Linda's depression and significant job stress (tenure-track junior faculty) actually caused me to seek the care of a psychologist. This eventually resulted in Linda entering therapy. ... I learned two things from my brief course of therapy that were of significant comfort to me. One, I did not cause Linda's depression. ... Two, I cannot fix Linda's depression. No amount of love will result in a cure. Realizing this ... [has] allowed me to continue to care for my wife, but not to be consumed by her illness. Essentially, I have given myself permission to avoid having my own life destroyed by depression. This has resulted in a much better degree of communication and honesty between my wife and myself and, strange as it sounds, our marriage is actually stronger now that I "care" less. I would bet that spouses and children of depressed people have as diverse a group of stories as the depressed themselves.

Even with letters of this kind, it took reading a wonderful book by Arthur Frank to get me thinking seriously that *Speaking of Sadness* told only half an important story.[9] Frank's book *The Wounded Storyteller* is about the need of ill people to tell their narratives as a way of reconstructing the "map of their lives." His thesis is that storytelling is a way to create order from the chaos generated by serious illness. At an early point, Frank, who previously had written a book on his experience with cancer, explores the social nature of all illness narratives since they presume an audience of some sort.[10] An illness narrative is told *to someone*. There really is no such thing as a self-story because stories are inherently social productions. That is, all self-stories are really self–other stories. In the concluding paragraph of his first chapter, Frank makes the following observation about those who bear witness to and try to help sick people:

> The voices of the ill are easy to ignore, because these voices are often faltering in tone and mixed in message. ... These voices bespeak conditions ... that most of us would rather forget our vulnerability to. Listening is hard, but it is also a fundamentally moral act. ... [I]n listening for the other, we listen for ourselves. The moment of

witness in the story crystallizes a mutuality of need, when each is *for* the other.[11]

Throughout his book Frank examines the difficult relationship between sufferers of any illness and those who care about them. Anyone who cares for a sick person becomes implicated in their sickness. In this way, as affirmed by Leslie's story and by my Midwestern Internet acquaintance, all illnesses are potentially contagious in the sense that the stories of sick people become deeply woven into the biographies of those who feel a commitment to them.[12] Our social connections are secured by the stories we tell each other about our lives; they are the medium through which lives become intertwined. Recently, I read the same idea expressed in Lauren Slater's eloquent book about mental illness called *Welcome to My Country*. Slater writes, "I don't know at what point one can call a story truly one's own, where the boundaries between one mind and another meet. . . . Perhaps narratives are the one realm that cannot ever . . . be confidently claimed by any individual."[13]

As I read Frank's descriptions of the kinds of narratives told by wounded storytellers, I kept thinking about *wounded listeners*. It's not that this was the first time I had considered the difficulties of those who must listen to sick people or observe their travail. At several points in *Speaking of Sadness* I wondered about the effects of my own depression on my family. Early in the book I wrote, "I have worried a great deal over the last two decades about the influence on my children, a son now 23 and a daughter 20, of growing up in a household with a father who was often unreasonable, crazily irritable, and too often inaccessible. It is also nearly astounding that my wife has not left me." Still, the plight of those who listen, watch, and try to help emotionally ill people had been only at the periphery of my thinking.

The publication of *Speaking of Sadness* influenced my life in another unanticipated way that sensitized me to the circumstances of those who feel obliged to listen to sad tales of emotional distress. People who know my work sometimes seek me out for conversation about their troubles, believing, I suppose, that I have some kind of special expertise to share. As the author of a book on depression, I have been unexpectedly cast into the listener role. These recent experiences have made me evaluate, if only as a practical matter, my moral obligations to those who wish me to hear their stories.

To appreciate the contours of my new listening role, consider my relationship with Helen, one of my undergraduate students. Helen became my advisee a few years ago and over time we came to share parts of our lives. Discussions about themes in *Speaking of Sadness* led eventually to confessions about her own long-term emotional distress, pain she only recently could name as depression. Although I made it perfectly clear that I am not a therapist, I was still somewhat worried about having crossed the always unclear teacher/student boundary. Still, I enjoyed the conversation because Helen is bright and had interesting things to say about illness and because she expressed gratitude for being able to freely share her thoughts. The shift from the democracy of intellectual talk about emotional pain to my more purely listening role followed the downhill slope of Helen's love relationship at the time. The process of her breakup with a boyfriend precipitated her emotional breakdown.

As things grew worse Helen began to see a psychiatrist and shortly thereafter started on a "trial" of psychotropic drugs. Rather than reducing my contact with her, Helen's encounter with her doctor and the "medical model" of mental illness only generated a barrage of questions about pills, biology, and psychiatry. If her concerns were exclusively the product of confusion about, say, the meaning of taking antidepressant medications, it would not have been especially difficult to meet her needs. Increasingly, though, Helen's unfolding narrative was of the sort that Arthur Frank has called a "chaos story." Chaos stories are the hardest to listen to because there is no rational thread to them—they are constituted by a flood of feelings that words inevitably fail to express. "The teller of chaos stories is, preeminently, the wounded storyteller. . . .

The person living the chaos story has no distance from her life and no reflective grasp on it. Lived chaos makes reflection, and consequently story telling, impossible. . . . [T]hese stories cannot literally be told but can only be lived."[14]

On many days Helen would appear at my office door early in the morning after another sleepless night, looking drawn and literally shaking with anxiety. In that state she would tell me, "I feel like I'll go crazy if I'm alone today. I just can't bear to be alone." Such moments require decisions and mine was to let her camp out in my office for a few hours until she calmed down. In making this decision I had to somehow balance our conversational history, our teacher/student relationship, my compassion for her pain, the immediacy of her needs, and my faculty responsibilities. Most of the time I felt that the choice to allow use of my office as a haven, as a refuge, was the right one.

I sometimes marvel at the fact that after dealing with depression for more than two decades, spending years going to therapists of one sort or another, and then writing a book on the subject, I can think of little else to do but listen in the face of another person's pain. I may know more than others about regularities in the depression experience, but I have no great wisdom, no magic words to pass along to people like my student Helen. When she tried to choke out the circumstances of her life that were making her so miserable, I felt paralyzed. Comments meant to comfort—"Just try to hang in there. It *does* get better."—sounded inane to me even as I said the words.

The combination of personal reflection, communications from family and friends of sick people, books on the experience of illness, and my own bewilderment about how best to respond to others in emotional pain strengthened my conviction that caregivers to mentally ill persons have important, untold stories to tell. I decided that one additional way to test the prospects for a book on the subject would be to return to a self-help group that I had attended regularly a few years back.

Although most of those attending the weekly meetings of

the Manic Depressive and Depressive Association (MDDA) are victims of depression or manic-depression, there is an affiliated "Family and Friends" group. I hoped that because I had previously been an MDDA member and, more recently, had been a guest speaker, that the Family and Friends group would let me attend as an observer.[15] Happily, they said "yes" to my proposal and I have been a regular in the group for more than three years. The stories I hear in this forum absolutely astonish me because of their sheer poignancy, courage, and drama. Even after completing the work for this book, I have maintained my ties with the group because I now view several of the people there as friends and because I want to know how they are faring in their ongoing struggle to help a parent, child, spouse, or sibling with a disastrous life condition.

At first, I just felt overwhelmed at hearing the details of each person's account. On any given evening I might hear about the unimaginable pain surrounding the decision to have a child removed from one's home by the police, the powerlessness of visiting a spouse or child in a hospital who is so muddled by powerful medications that he or she can barely speak, the shame that accompanies hating someone you love because of what their illness has done to you and your family, the guilt that lingers from the belief that you might somehow be responsible for another person's descent into mental illness, the confusion associated with navigating the Byzantine complexities of the mental health system, the fear associated with waiting for the next phone call announcing yet another suicide attempt by someone close to you, the disappointment that a talented son or daughter may never realize even a fraction of their potential, the exhaustion that accompanies full-time caregiving, or the frustration of being unable to take even a brief vacation. Pain, powerlessness, shame, guilt, confusion, fear, disappointment, exhaustion, frustration: these emotions are the currency of conversation among the Family and Friends group members.

Whatever might be the distinctiveness of their individual circumstances, the twenty-five or so regulars at each week's meetings are struggling with the same underlying concerns. They come to find solace in the company of others who understand their agony, to share coping strategies, and to gird themselves for the inevitable bouts with the mental illness monster. Underneath all this is the matter of responsibility. Nearly always during the two-hour meeting, someone is asked to recite what I now think of as the group's "Four Cs Mantra." Heads nod when one or another member says these familiar words: "I didn't cause it. I can't control it. I can't cure it. All I can do is cope with it." These are folks trying to incorporate the wisdom of the Four Cs into their daily lives. I say "trying" because however many times the Four Cs are invoked, they stand in contrast to the stories that precede and follow their recitation. All agree that they need to find ways to cope. However, as each member's tale unfolds, it is also unmistakably filled with doubt about the storyteller's role in causing, controlling, and curing a loved one's depression or mania.

Listening every week to the circumstances of the support group members persuaded me that the case of mental illness poses distinctive caregiving contingencies. Although chronic and life-threatening illnesses of any sort will generate confusion, ambiguity, complexity, and anxiety about setting proper boundaries with a sick person, these problems are compounded in the case of mental illness. For example, rarely will patients question the diagnosis of such serious physical illnesses as cancer or heart disease. In contrast, those diagnosed with depression, manic-depression, or schizophrenia often vigorously deny the disease label. Unlike most physical illnesses, caregivers to the mentally ill (especially parents) must often contend with the possibility that they are somehow implicated in the creation of the other's problem. Finally, despite their best efforts, caregivers are sometimes treated as though they were an enemy by their loved one. In these ways, mental illness poses problems of greater interpretive complexity for caregivers than even the most tragic physical illnesses.

In some respects, each individual story I have heard over the last three years, either in the Family and Friends group or tape-recorded one-on-one, is unique. Mental illness takes multiple forms and disrupts family life in countless ways. No doubt, the person telling each story also feels that no one in the world knows precisely what they are going through, and they are right in that feeling. Everyone in pain is, in an existential sense, alone with it. No one can actually feel another individual's pain; all they can do is imagine it. At the same time, a sociological angle of vision presumes that there are consistencies and uniformities in even the most personally chaotic life experiences.[16] The explicit content of each person's caregiving narrative might be different, but their experiences, I want to argue, display common, underlying forms.

In the last decade or so, a number of personal memoirs about mental illness have been published. Most of these books[17] recount what it is like to be ill, but, recently, family members of emotionally ill persons have begun to tell their stories.[18] As valuable as these accounts are, they can only hint at features of caregiving that transcend the particularities of a single case. The great advantage of my three years of listening in a self-help group and then systematically analyzing sixty lengthy interviews is that such a methodology lets me see overarching and repeating themes, patterns, or social forms in all the cases.

Kai Erikson provides a nice example for illustrating how a sociological perspective is necessary to see social patterns that would be missed if we only look at things "up close and personal," as they used to say on *Wide World of Sports*.[19] He has us imagine that we are walking along 42nd Street near Times Square. At the street level we can clearly see the faces of thousands of people who pass us. We can see their individual expressions, their particular body idioms, their apparent ages, and so on. At this range, they normally appear to take no notice of anyone around them. Each stranger appears as a solitary atom, buzzing along in a thoroughly independent way.

Were we, however, to climb to the roof of a nearby twelve-story building and look down on the flow of sidewalk traffic, we would see an extraordinary thing. It is true that from this vantage point we miss the specifics of each individual. We would, though, witness a miraculous pattern—thousands of people moving along the street in an incredibly well-organized, efficient, and cooperative fashion. Moreover, each person on the street would likely be wholly unaware of their contribution to the web of behavior necessary to sustain such an enormously complex social order. It is as if each pedestrian is guided by an invisible social force, a kind of social gravity, about which they have only the vaguest awareness. I am proposing that most persons grappling with someone else's suffering, like street pedestrians, are only dimly aware of how widespread, shared, and culturally prescribed are their feelings about caregiving, feelings that they imagine are unique and incomparable.

The story that began this chapter is absolutely distinctive in its details. Yet, as the following chapters will show, Leslie's account also displays social processes, emotions, confusions, and challenges that cut across the sixty interviews I conducted for this book. Like all the caregivers who will speak in the pages to come, Leslie engaged in ongoing interpretations of how to "draw the line" between herself and Mike, her son. Having spoken with her recently, I know that Leslie is still trying to find a workable balance of involvement and distance in her son's life. Her account also illustrates that the need to care is propelled by emotions of both obligation and love. The shortened version of her caregiving biography strongly hints that parents feel a different combination of love and responsibility than do spouses, siblings, or the children of mentally ill people. As well, the disruption in her marriage caused by Mike's illness suggests that men and women create a different calculus of caregiving. Finally, like everyone I interviewed, Leslie had to learn how to navigate within a set of complicated mental health bureaucracies.

The Burden of Sympathy is organized around the central, repeating, and common dimensions that I was able to discern in my interviews with caregivers. In large measure, the boundaries of my writing are determined by the accounts of my informants. I have tried to organize my materials to best capture the shared features of their experiences. I expect that caregivers who read this book will see their own lives reflected in the stories of others. If I have done my work well—if I have been a good sociological guide—the analysis of interview materials in each chapter will provide readers with new perspectives on their own caregiving struggles. In a fashion, I see this whole enterprise as a storytelling venture. I can only offer my theoretical accounts in the chapters to follow because I have had the good fortune to hear so many compelling stories like Leslie's. That being so, let me conclude this first chapter by briefly describing the blueprint I have in mind for telling you how I have made sense of their narratives.

Chapter 2, "Bearing Responsibility," elaborates the interpretive task most essentially connecting all sixty people with whom I spoke. All caregivers must somehow negotiate the dialectic of closeness and distance with an ill person. They puzzle about how best to "draw the line" between themselves and a sick person. The guiding question for Chapter 2 asks, "What features of the situation do family members take into account as they try to construct boundaries of obligation between themselves and the mentally ill person in their lives?" As throughout this book, I conceive the relationship between caregivers and patients in processual terms. The way caregivers think about their obligations shifts over the course of their "joint career" with the ill person.

I identify four interpretive junctures in the evolution of caregivers' consciousness about responsibility. They move through an initial period of learning about the illness and hoping for a quick resolution. Those new to mental illness and the caregiving role rely heavily on doctors to solve what they hope will be a limited and curable problem. Caregivers must, however, eventually confront the reality that a loved one's illness will not disappear. This recognition generates new expectations for themselves and the person in their care. At a point, nearly everyone interviewed reassessed how much responsibility ill persons must themselves bear for their own condition. If, as the Puritans believed, "God helps those who help themselves," caregivers eventually adopt a secularized version of that dictum—"Caregivers should help only patients willing to help themselves." Finally, respondents often reach a critical moment when they must decide whether their own health and identities have become so compromised that they can no longer maintain a commitment to care.

Chapter 3, "Managing Emotions," continues the themes of the previous chapter. Just as there are predictable changes in feelings of responsibility over time, the interviews reveal comparable and patterned transformations in caregivers' emotions. Although sociologists have always understood feelings of obligation, responsibility, and duty to be the moral cornerstones of society, little attention has been given to the ways such feelings are evoked, interpreted, managed, and acted on in everyday life. Every respondent in this study felt the emotions of fear, confusion, hope, compassion, sympathy, love, frustration, sadness, grief, anger, resentment, and guilt. However, there are consistent changes in the relative subjective significance and intensity of each of these emotions over time.

Prior to a firm medical diagnosis, caregivers experience what I call "emotional anomie." They are fundamentally confused by the behaviors of a family member and quite simply don't know precisely what to feel. Such anomie reflects the sheer bewilderment of a life that has moved rapidly from coherence and predictability to chaos and disorder. Eventually, a diagnosis of depression, manic-depression, or schizophrenia provides a medical frame that clarifies the circumstance of caregivers and provokes feelings of hope, compassion, and sympathy. At a certain point, initial optimism that their loved one's mental illness can be fixed gives way to a sense of its likely permanence. The frame of permanence, coupled with doubts about the ill person's inability to control their objectionable behaviors, ushers in more negative feelings of anger, resentment, even hate. Some of the respondents eventually conclude that none of their efforts can successfully change things. Such a recognition can sometimes lead to an acceptance of the other's condition. Acceptance, in turn, liberates caregivers from the earlier burdensome belief that it is their duty to somehow solve the problem.

One of the most essential ideas in social psychology is that a person's various statuses influence how he or she defines and experiences the world. In Chapter 4, "Family Ties," my goal is to show how feelings of obligation are tied to one's "social location" within the family—as parent, child, sibling, or spouse. This chapter also departs from the style of data presentation in Chapters 2 and 3. Although allowing lots of people to speak is an effective way to display caregiving commonalties, it is also important to provide you with a fuller sense of caregivers' lives. Thus, in Chapter 4, I will describe three "case histories." To complement Leslie's narrative—a mother's story—I want to introduce you to three other people whose interviews reflect the distinctive experiences of children, siblings, and spouses.

Jason's mother had her first psychotic break when he was seven or eight. His is a story of childhood terror and feelings of betrayal by a father who he believes did not sufficiently protect him. Now, as a thirty-year-old, Jason is still trying to heal from the sense of abandonment that inevitably arises when children cannot count on parents to nurture them. Angie still mourns the alleged suicide of her brother four years before we spoke. Her account highlights a sister's struggle to decide just how much she owed to her chronically ill brother, her aging parents, and herself. Finally, I'll tell Gail's story. Shortly into their five-year marriage, Gail's husband was diagnosed with manic-depression. Although she remains firm in her resolve to help the man she loves, Gail must also contemplate the circumstances that would justify leaving her marriage.

I earlier mentioned that the members of the Family and Friends support group I attend each week share an illness ideology of sorts. The Four Cs have it that caregivers did not cause the problem, can't cure it, have no control over it, and can only cope with it. In Chapter 5, I examine more closely the first three Cs—cause, control, and cure. Although group members appear largely to embrace the Four Cs, it is quite another thing to honestly believe that they had absolutely no role in causing it and that they can do nothing to cure or, at least, control a spouse's, child's, parent's, or sibling's illness. My examination of cause, cure, and control, so central to the talk of caregivers, proceeds from the observation that all human beings must create theories about significant features of their lives. Just as we construct theories about such matters as parenting, education, crime, and falling in love, caregivers must construct a usable theory about the causes of mental illness and how best to respond to it. In Chapter 5, I describe how the people I interviewed try to create practically useful theories about cause, cure, and control.

The fourth C is coping. In a fashion, every chapter in this book is about the efforts of family caregivers to maintain personal equilibrium as they deal with the horrible fallout from another person's mental illness. However, the data and analysis throughout the first five chapters center largely on the day-to-day, face-to-face relationships of ill people and family caregivers. In Chapter 6, "Surviving the System," my analysis shifts as I am more self-consciously guided by the simple sociological truth that all of us are bounded by social structures that powerfully structure our lives. To live in a society means to be embedded within a dense network of institutions that shape our choices and often literally affect our "life chances."[20] A catastrophic mental illness propels sick people and their families into the mental health system. Suddenly, caregivers must cope with police, the court system, social workers, doctors, hospital administrators, government agencies, and insurance companies. Rather than diminishing their pain and confusion, the system too often bewilders and marginalizes family members.

Chapter 6 follows the joint "institutional careers" of patients and families. As in other chapters, careful reading of the interview materials suggests a sequential process. At some point it becomes undeniably clear that a person is in terrible trouble, that there is a full-blown crisis to manage. If an ill person refuses treatment, the crisis may require family members to seek the "help" of community crisis teams, the police, and the court system. Every person interviewed for this book cared for a child, spouse, sibling, or parent who eventually required hospitalization. Although providing them initial relief, caregivers soon discovered that hospitalization would not solve the problem. Hospitalization also meant entering the domain of professional "experts." Caregivers often felt ignored by psychiatrists whose therapeutic perspective typically did not extend to family caregivers. Finally, nearly every person I interviewed expressed anger about the incredible difficulties in securing private insurance or government benefits. Chapter 6, therefore, expands on the system-related tasks of managing crises, negotiating hospital bureaucracies, dealing with doctors, and finding ways to pay for treatment.

Throughout this first chapter I have been claiming that the subject matter for this volume permits exploration of such essential questions as: "What do we owe each other?" "What are the moral boundaries of family relationships?" "To what extent are we bound to care for each other?" "What are the limits of sympathy in dealing with another person's trouble?" "What social contingencies impinge on our responsibilities and obligations to each other?" Such questions could not be any more fundamental to the sociological enterprise since inquiry into the nature of social obligations is tantamount to asking "How is society possible?"[21] Reasonable approaches to these questions cannot, however, be divorced from history and social structure since, as C. W. Mills noted over forty years ago, "the biographies of men and women, the kinds of individuals they variously become cannot be understood without reference to the historical structures in which the milieus of their everyday lives are organized. Historical transformations carry meanings not only for individual ways of life, but for the very character—the limits and possibilities of the human being."[22]

The last chapter, "Caring in Postmodern America," departs from the interview data and offers a general argument about how the distinctive values of contemporary American society, in contrast to earlier historical eras, shape our consciousness about caring for others in trouble. I consider how the imperatives of the so-called "postmodern" world impinge on the possibilities of deep and caring human bonds, how the progressive loosening of social bonds in

America may have diminished our felt obligations toward people who are suffering from all kinds of ills.

Certainly, available sociological writing on America's ethic of individualism provides ammunition to argue that social connections, and thus social obligations, are becoming increasingly loose and nonbinding.[23] Some observers, like my colleague Charles Derber, view rampant individualism as a kind of social virus that has for decades been eroding America's national character.[24] Early in his book *The Wilding of America* Derber describes the Ik, a Ugandan people studied by the anthropologist Colin Turnbull about twenty years ago. The Ik, living in a hostile physical, economic, and political environment, have become a loveless people for whom personal morality does not extend beyond crass self-preservation. Because each person in Ik society regards every other person, even family members, as competitors for scarce resources, they have thoroughly lost all capacity for empathy with the suffering of others. It would be melodramatic to identify Americans too closely with the Ik, but perhaps we are a people who have become more Ik-like.

In contrast to those apocalyptic visions that see America's ethic of expressive individualism as eradicating empathy, I feel that the accounts of the sixty people interviewed for this book allow a more optimistic view. With a few exceptions, my conversations were with people who have "hung in there." Their route has been chaotic, unspeakably painful, and often damaging to their own physical and emotional health. Still, they have thus far stayed the course! Precisely because of their commitment, some readers, and I imagine fellow sociologists, will complain that these folks are unrepresentative. They might say that these days the more typical response of American family members confronted by severe mental illness is to withdraw emotionally or "cut out" altogether. Of course, there are no good statistics to tell us just how representative a sample I have. Let's imagine, though, that those who speak in later chapters are unlike most Americans in their dedication to an emotionally ill family member. I say, "All the more reason to study them!"

Robert Bogdan and Steven Taylor, affiliated with the Center on

Human Policy at Syracuse University, have been calling for a "so-ciology of acceptance." They point out that "for a quarter century sociologists have concentrated on stigma and the labeling and re-jection of people with negatively valued physical, mental, and be-havioral difference."[25] While Bogdan and Taylor do not dispute that "deviant" people are often silenced, abandoned, and shunted off to the margins of society, their studies of profoundly disabled people reveal that there are some people who form genuine, deep, loving, and enduring friendships with them. They argue that it is *precisely* because intimate, accepting ties between "normal" people and those with profound disabilities are uncommon that they ought to be studied. By learning about the basis for social acceptance when we might not expect it, we may be better able to foster it. Similarly, I hope that by showing how the individuals I studied continued to care under difficult circumstances, it will make it easier for others, faced with mental illness at home, to do so also.

Aside from providing the blueprint for this book, Chapter 1 has stressed the importance of life stories because of their potential to transform both the storyteller and the listener. In a truly lovely and moving memoir recounting his lifelong relationship with his brother Robert, who has spent most of the last thirty years in and out of psychiatric hospitals, Jay Neugeboren explains what kept him at the task of writing their joint story. He puts it this way:

> I'm not interested in writing about [Robert's] life in order to exploit him or embarrass him, to find villains or designate blame, to come up with answers to how and why he's led the life he's led, or to what mental illness is or is not and what we can do about it, but in order—simply and most of all—to tell his story as best I can, and thereby be a witness to his life, in all its complexity, uniqueness, hope, and despair—in all, that is, that makes it fully human.... As painful and grim as any experience, or any life may be, to be able to transform it into story, like the act of remembering ... can offer us a kind of consolation—and, sometimes, of joy—unlike any other.[26]

This book relies on lengthy conversations with people who have shared the double story of someone close to them with a mental illness and their own efforts to stand by them. Of course, it is practically impossible to know where one story leaves off and the other begins because the two become so bound together. Many of the people with whom I spoke thanked me for the opportunity to tell their stories, often expressing that there is a healing and new understanding that comes from articulating their experiences.

I'm glad that the research work I do allows a kind of catharsis for many of the people who shared such personal and difficult parts of their biographies. I consider their stories as precious gifts. And precisely because there is a sacredness to what they have told me, I have felt a special obligation as a writer to use their narratives in a way that honestly conveys the complexity, courage, heroism, and humanity associated with caring for someone with a mental illness. I know that listening to their accounts has vastly deepened my understanding of what it means to maintain commitments. I hope that I have honored their stories by using them in a way that expands your capacity for empathy, tolerance, and caring.

TWO

Bearing Responsibility

I just did it because that's what I was supposed to do.
... What the hell are you supposed to do if you have
a sick parent in the house ... and you're part of the
family? ... What are you supposed to do, throw them
by the wayside? ... I mean, I love my parents. ... I did
it out of love and caring and [as] a son who was, you
know, the oldest.

EDUCATION ADMINISTRATOR, *age forty-three, son*

I know ... my limit is reached [when] all I think about
is ... getting her [mother] in the car and driving off a
cliff because I can't stand to be with her and I feel she
can't do this to people anymore. ... In a way my identity disappeared because I was just sucked into that
blackness and weirdness.

INSURANCE ADMINISTRATOR,
age forty-six, daughter/sister

When Nancy announced that she and her husband were actually
finalizing plans for a two-week vacation to Florida, her Family and
Friends supporters spontaneously applauded. The topic of vacations, Nancy's in particular, was often discussed in the MDDA
group. The conversation was always about the difficulty family
members had in leaving home, even for a week or so, because they
couldn't stop worrying about what might happen in their absence.
Parents tried to persuade each other that since they could not stop
their ill children from unraveling even when close by, they logically

ought to be able to go on vacation. However, many, like Nancy, could not bring themselves to do it. In those conversations Nancy often expressed the group's collective sentiment when she said, "I would never forgive myself if anything were to happen while I was gone." Like others, Nancy had real cause for worry. Her forty-two-year-old daughter had been first hospitalized two years earlier after a suicide attempt left her comatose. Diane survived, although with brain damage, and, still suicidal, has been in a hospital ever since. At age seventy-two, Nancy is especially distraught because "these are the years that, you know, were supposed to be our good years, and she has totally destroyed them."

Nancy was among the first persons I interviewed for the book. After hearing bits and pieces about her life, I was not surprised that she lived in a well-kept, modest, middle-class neighborhood. Her home was small, but obviously maintained with great care and love. It turned out that her husband Frank was there, and Nancy asked whether he might join our conversation. I was glad to talk with both of them since experience has taught me that valuable insight often comes from interchanges between spouses during an interview. After we finished our interview, Nancy and Frank gave me a tour of their home. They were especially proud of an addition that Frank had built himself. It had been a separate apartment for Diane, who lived with them before she tried to take her life. They hoped that she would one day be back, but this seemed unlikely because of the seriousness of her illness. It was also unlikely since, as I learned during our talk, Diane's psychiatrist did not want her returning home, believing strongly that she needs to gain independence from her parents.

Individuals are always eager to convey in detail those parts of their stories that most essentially define events for them. These symbolically powerful themes give each interview a distinctive flavor, tone, or motif. My talk with Nancy and Frank centered on Nancy's struggle to "let go" of her daughter, to loosen her emotional bond with Diane. The trauma of the previous two years, conversations with Diane, and consultation with her doctors persuaded Nancy that "if Diane is going to survive I've got to let her go and the only way I can let her go is not to have her here." Nancy's problem, though, as reflected in the vacation issue, is that she simply can't let go; her heart won't cooperate. Throughout the interview she offered small details that helped me to understand her difficulty in drawing firmer boundaries between herself and Diane. For example, a ritual has evolved that requires Nancy to sit by the phone each day, waiting for her daughter's call. She would like to be freed of this obligation, but so far cannot sever even this thin thread. When I gently pushed her to explain why she found it so difficult to make even a modest change in the telephone routine, she told me:

> Letting go to me would be having the phone ring at ten minutes past nine in the morning and not answering and saying [to myself], "I'm not going to talk with her this morning." But would I be able to do it? I don't know. And if I tried it, then I would feel guilty the rest of the day, because if she called back at one o'clock and she had been sick, I'd never forgive myself for not having talked to her. . . . I know what's needed, but, you know, in my heart I can't do it. . . . I'm very aware that [the bond] needs to be broken, but either I don't want to or I can't. One or the other. And I think basically it's that I don't want to.

Nancy and Frank did finally take their vacation. They "checked in every few days just to make sure that everything was all right." When she returned to the Family and Friends group, everyone wanted to know how things went. More congratulations were offered to Nancy for taking such a big step in gaining a measure of control over her own life. The conversation about Nancy's triumph lingered because everyone understood it as an object lesson. Whether or not they worry about taking vacations, everyone I have heard talk in the group and in my interviews is trying to find a healthy balance between involvement and distance in their relationship with an ill family member. All of them would agree with

Nancy who, at several points, during our interview said, "I think the hardest part [of caregiving] is not knowing whether what you are doing is right or wrong." This chapter focuses on the central theme of Nancy's interview—indeed, of this whole enterprise. I examine how the people interviewed assess the nature of their obligations to ill children, spouses, parents, or brothers and sisters.

My analysis throughout this chapter is directed at understanding what family members take into account as they try to set obligation boundaries between themselves and the mentally ill person in their lives. Both my theoretical approach[1] and the data collected requires that we understand caregivers' assessments about proper involvement[2] with a mentally ill person as *a process over time*. It is a process characterized by intense efforts to make sense of another's illness and to negotiate how best to help them without becoming engulfed by their misery.[3] I will show that the kinds of boundaries that seem appropriate at the outset of an illness are quite different from those established at later points in a caregiver's evolving "joint career" with an ill person.[4]

As is so frequently the case when analyzing qualitative data, the central metaphor that animates my thinking comes from the words of the respondents themselves. With extraordinary regularity, the people interviewed spoke about their difficulty in *drawing the line* between themselves and an ill spouse, child, brother, or parent. We learn from their comments that decisions about how and where to draw responsibility lines are surrounded by intense emotions, equivocation, uncertainty, and ambivalence. Along with the kind of bewilderment and consternation intrinsic to relationships with mentally ill people, decisions about how to draw boundaries are compounded by a widely held cultural prescription that over-involvement with dependent people might properly be considered a disease. The existence of a whole social movement in America dedicated to avoiding "enabling" and "codependence" is striking evidence of Americans' confusion about the permissible limits of human closeness.[5] Co-dependency can arise as a pathological condition only in a society that fosters deep ambivalence about the value of extensive ties.

This chapter, then, is primarily about how sixty people draw and then redraw appropriate boundaries between themselves and a sick family member. Their stories attest to the near impossibility of arriving at a line that makes sense and is workable over time. Eventually, respondents reluctantly realize that whatever line they draw, like the proverbial line in the sand, is transitory and easily blown away by the shifting and wholly unpredictable winds of mental illness. Still, unless they abandon the relationship altogether, family members have no alternative in the face of another's emotional illness except to try over and again to find a balance between the requirements of care and the maintenance of their own well-being. My goal is to reveal regularities in caretakers' thinking, feeling, and behaving as they try to determine an appropriate level of commitment to an ill person. The question directing my analysis in the following pages asks, "What features of the situation do family members take into account as they try to construct boundaries of obligation between themselves and the mentally ill person in their lives?"

The interview materials suggest four overlapping dimensions that frame the relationship between caregivers and family members. While each of these four experiential moments generally occurs sequentially, it would be a mistake to understand them as operating in an absolutely stage-like fashion. Rather, I view these interpretive junctures in family members' illness careers as bearing a simultaneous, dialectical, and mutually transformative relationship with each other. I offer them as a framework for economically presenting the data and, thus, for looking at key elements of consciousness shared by nearly all the respondents in this study. They are:

1. HOPING AND LEARNING—Those new to mental illness and the caregiver role rely heavily on medicine to solve what they hope will be a limited and curable problem in the life of a loved one.

2. REVISING EXPECTATIONS—Most caregivers must eventually confront the reality that a loved one's mental illness will not disappear. This recognition, in turn, generates new expectations for both the sick family member and themselves.

3. ASSESSING RESPONSIBILITY—A critical factor in determining their degree of obligation is caregivers' ongoing assessment of how much responsibility a sick person can and ought to take in solving their own problem.

4. PRESERVING ONESELF—At critical junctures during the course of caregiving, respondents grapple with having to decide whether their own health and identities are so compromised that they can no longer maintain a commitment to care.

Drawing the Line

Eventually, as later sections will show, caregivers do withdraw support under certain predictable circumstances. However, as they recount their histories of caring when a family member becomes mentally ill, they nearly uniformly felt a strong obligation to care at the outset of the "trouble." Here's a sampling of the way they saw their obligations early in their caregiving careers:

I don't really see what I am doing as duty. . . . I mean, I know that I have a duty to make it through the snow storm to work on a bad day. I see that as duty. I see that as being a good soldier. . . . I won't let you down, and that kind of thing. I don't think any of those thoughts in relation to being here for him [son]. I just feel that it is very much an unfinished job. . . . Responsibility is deeper [than duty]. Duty—you know exactly the limits of it. . . . Responsibility, it's your essence. I mean, could you sleep? Could your soul rest? Would your dreams be troubled if you really didn't meet your responsibility.

RETIRED BOOK EDITOR, *age fifty-one, mother*

↪

My mother looks at it that I should take care of her. . . . You know . . . "I gave birth to her, so she owes me this life (of hers)." . . . So, you know, it's one of those things. You make the decision. I guess you allow yourself to feel the obligation. Because I could walk away from it . . . but I look at it that when I go to meet my God, I don't want to have any feeling . . . like I didn't do everything that I could have.

ACCOUNTANT, *age thirty-five, daughter*

↩

I felt like I owed her that, like I should take care of her. You know, she is my mom and I felt . . . I mean I don't know if it was her saying it to me or me feeling it as well. I mean, I guess when I was growing up . . . what I saw was my mom always taking care of other people and doing things for other people in our family. So as a child, I mean, you definitely learn these things, you know? By example, you see that, okay, this is how the world works. . . . You know, my mom is doing things for her mom or her relatives and, you know, it's just natural.[6]

RESEARCH ASSISTANT, *age twenty-three, daughter*

Although Chapter 4 will elaborate the issue, I should note here that the cultural mandate to care for an ill family member is not felt equally by everyone. The sociologist Candace Clark has made important observations about the connection between the social statuses of persons and the "width" of their respective sympathy margins.[7] Spouses, for example, are expected to honor sympathy requests for problems that would seem too trivial in another relationship. Husbands and wives can complain to each other at length about a bad day at work, for example, and feel wronged if their partner does not pay close attention and extend considerable sympathy. The relationships between parents and children are bounded by quite different rules. In this case, the margins are asymmetrical since parents are expected to freely extend far more sympathy to their children (especially, of course, young children) than they can legitimately expect in return. In particular, mothers of sick children clearly expressed the greatest obligation to care.

We bring these children into the world. We give them life. We're responsible. Until the day God takes them, we are their parents, we are responsible, and no matter what. If there is an illness there, you have an extra responsibility. I really believe that and I feel that with all my heart.

REAL ESTATE BROKER, *age forty-five, mother*

⤳

It has got to be heartbreaking to see your kid in a mental hospital.

I wanted to kill myself, David, I wanted to kill myself. Do you understand that? It wasn't just because I was depressed. It was because I felt responsible and helpless to do anything and no one loved him but me in the whole wide world and my love wasn't enough. I couldn't put my arms around him and give him what he needed. I wanted to die. . . . I mean, I tried to bargain with God, "Take my life, fix my kid's." To this day, if God said to me, "Will you come with me now if I make them all happy and straightened out and productive and they will be all right?" I'll go, "Yes! Gladly!" You know, "[If I] never have another moment's happiness. Fine! I'll go with you!"

UNEMPLOYED, *age fifty, mother*

Although it is utterly devastating to have a child become mentally ill, several mothers nevertheless acknowledged that it would be difficult to give up the caregiving role. In one case, a mother of a child who recently became eighteen explained that she was about to experience a deep identity loss because her daughter, in the throes of a manic episode, planned to leave home against her wishes.

Oh my God, how do I be her mother [now]? How do I be her mother when she is not living in my house? And now that she's hit the road, it's a real crisis for me. . . . I had to give up the last piece of managing her life. She's eighteen and I have no more to say. And she hit the

road. And . . . she's not safe. . . . As long as she was in my sphere . . .
I was going to manage it. . . . I can't do it anymore. I don't know
what to do with myself. I don't know how to be her mother [now].
From the day she was born she didn't eat and didn't sleep and she
needed fifteen casts and had diarrhea, and all that stuff. I've been
doing that (caring for her) since the day she was born, eighteen years
plus three weeks.

PHYSICAL THERAPY TEACHER, *age forty-nine, mother*

Men appear to have a different perspective on caregiving. This
"finding" fits with the frequently made observation that women
have always been socialized to be caregivers and feel far more comfortable with that role than men. Deborah Tannen argues that when
it comes to human relations problems, men are solution-oriented
whereas women are sympathy-oriented.[8] Men sometimes quickly
"burn out" as caregivers. Women, on the other hand, who do not
typically approach their commitment to a sick family member in
solution terms, are, compared to men, normally more tolerant caregivers. Women, in other words, are often more involved caregivers
than men because they are trained for that role and because their
commitment to caregiving is not contingent on the eradication of
the problem. Women's words about obligation sometimes contrast
sharply with those of men, many of whom seem far more pragmatic
in determining the boundaries of their responsibilities. Two men,
for example, independently talked about how the travel demanded
by their work was a welcome respite from a home dominated by a
mentally ill partner or child.

I travel and that allows me some time alone with my thoughts . . . .
I think it helps. I enjoy . . . business trips. . . . I enjoyed it before I
really understood the full extent of my wife's disease, but it certainly
helps now. . . . My opinion [is that] this [mental illness] is something
guys handle better than women. . . . Guys are better at rationalizing
. . . [and] saying, "Yuh, I did do as good a job as I can. It wasn't a

great experience, but there wasn't anything else I could do about it and I've learned from it and then moved on."

SALESMAN, *age forty-two, husband*

↜

When I'm not around to take care of day-by-day issues, she's [wife] much stronger and much more able to do things on her own. I find when I'm away from home that I'm not worried because she seems to get her stuff together. So, I don't know to that extent whether my being there . . . helps her or gets in her way. I know when I travel for work—I tend to work eighteen-hour days—and, you know, go back to the hotel room when all the restaurants are closed and eat a box of crackers and peanut butter. So it's not a glamorous travel life but my mind tends to be at ease.

ELECTRONICS DESIGNER, *age sixty, husband*

This chapter began with the account of two elderly parents, Nancy and Frank, who are grappling with their daughter's illness. Nancy did most of the talking during the nearly three hours we spent together, but when Frank did speak it was largely to say that their health and enjoyment of life would be greatly enhanced if Nancy could succeed in gaining greater distance from their daughter. Each time Nancy expressed the feeling that it would be in everyone's best interest if her attachment to Diane were less, Frank seconded the emotion. Several times, Frank and Nancy acknowledged the sharp contrast in their respective attitudes about living a life more detached from Diane. Frank was better able than Nancy to "compartmentalize" different aspects of his life. Unlike Nancy, whose energy is so thoroughly absorbed by Diane's illness, Frank told me, "I bypass it. I concentrate on other things. I'll have something on the computer I want to do and I get my mind involved in that." At one point Nancy described Frank as an "escape artist." Here is a revealing string of conversation containing that "accusation":

NANCY: When we were talking [on the phone] she said: "This coming weekend you and daddy don't have to come up [to the hospital]. I'm not going to mind. You can have the weekend free."

KARP: So, what are you going to do?

NANCY: Probably nothing, just have the weekend to ourselves.

FRANK: I . . . feel liberated.

NANCY: Yeah, well, of course, you are the one doing the driving. . . . Several weeks ago I almost said to him, "Why don't I drive out and spend a couple of hours with Diane?" And I didn't say it because I figured if I said it once then he would say some weekend, "I really don't want to drive out." And I want him to be as much a part of our visiting her as mine is. You know, and I know he's tired. And I know that he resents it a little having to do it every weekend. But she is our child. We brought her into this world. It's up to us to take care of her while we are here.

FRANK: Yeah, well they're taking care of her out there.

NANCY: But we have to take care of her ourselves as mother and dad.

FRANK: We've gotta take care of ourselves.

NANCY: [*laughing*] See what I mean. . . . He's the escape artist. He goes downstairs to his computer. . . . Frank has always been able to shield himself.

FRANK: I always have something [to do]. In the past it was working in the garage, working on the cars, taking care of the lawn and all these [kinds of] things.

KARP: She just called you an escape artist. Is that an accurate description?

NANCY: Yes.

FRANK: It could be, yeah.

As Christena Nippert-Eng maintains in her provocative and insightful book about the linkages between work and home life, "All boundaries are socially constructed. . . . Over the natural non-order of things, we impose boundaries on everything, including our daily activities and the places and people with whom we pursue them."[9] Illness is surely a social occasion that sets in motion active efforts at "boundary work." Although any boundaries that human beings construct are subject to change and renegotiation over time, illness, because of its capacity to so thoroughly disrupt the coherence of

daily life, demands ongoing assessments about the proper boundaries between family caregivers and patients. Family members confronted with the reality of mental illness quickly learn that without
constructing appropriate boundaries they risk becoming engulfed
and potentially consumed by the other's illness. The inevitable task
that "well" family members face is to honor the obligation and
commitment they feel toward their sick spouse, parent, child, or
sibling without losing their own health and self.

As the following accounts will show, sustaining an appropriate
level of involvement with a mentally ill person is extraordinarily
difficult. Partly this is so because of the intrinsic nature of "mental"
illness. Not only is the course of the illness unpredictable, but the
ailing person may also act unpredictably. It is hard enough for a
healthy person to imagine the pain of a person who suffers from a
physical illness they themselves have never experienced. It is quite
another thing to understand a person who thinks and feels in ways
that seem totally incomprehensible. One respondent tried to draw
the contrast between the caregiving contingencies of physical and
mental illness this way:

> What do words mean? Words don't mean the same thing [to a
> mentally ill person]. Reality is not the same. You are not dealing in
> the same dimension. You have to understand . . . what that person's
> illness is and what the words really mean. . . . What frightens me
> about it is that reality is different. . . . Mentally ill people see things
> that are not there, or that I don't see, [that] other people don't see,
> and I don't know what they are seeing. I don't know what they are
> going to do. . . . Like my mother-in-law now has cancer [and] is
> having chemotherapy. She is a remarkable person. But there is like
> no problem. She is sick, she is tired. With the chemotherapy she is
> getting better. She is tired, she goes to sleep. She tells you, "I feel
> tired now" or "I don't feel like eating" or "I am sad I lost my hair."
> But we are all talking in the same place. She doesn't say, "I am sad
> that I lost my hair" and really mean that "I want to kill you and
> God is going to come down and strike everyone dead in this house

tonight." With a mentally ill person, you don't know. . . . I don't really feel like mentally ill people can hurt me. But . . . it's like you are just not in the same place and it makes me nervous. Like I really have no control.

INSURANCE ADMINISTRATOR, *age forty-six, daughter/sister*

The very unpredictability of the course of mental illness ensures that the lines established between caregiver and patient at one moment may not work shortly thereafter. Ill family members may, depending on their particular problem, alternate between episodes of deep depression, mania, florid psychosis, and wellness. Moreover, each discrete episode of illness may be different from those that preceded it. In the middle of an illness episode individuals may not comprehend their problem, may create huge difficulties in their own and caregivers' lives (such as spending money wildly, getting into automobile accidents, running away from home), and certainly may be incapable of expressing the sort of gratitude other ill people ordinarily extend to their caregivers. As a result, the central interpretive problem and practical dilemma for caregivers, heightened in the case of mental illness, is how to draw appropriate boundaries between themselves and a sick family member. The confusion, bewilderment, and consternation about "drawing the line" with someone suffering from depression, manic-depression, or schizophrenia is clear in the following comments:

The one [thing] that I think is the trickiest and is very emotional and very stressful is walking that line of "What do I do for this person, and what do I not do?" Because you constantly have to reevaluate that one. You know, you can hear yourself tell yourself [that] . . . you just have to do the best you can for this person, but it's sad and you try to accept that. But having to always say, "Now, what should I be doing for this person, and what should I not be doing? You know, they're disrupting my life. How much should I give?" It's a constant struggle. That's the one that's the toughest, and it just really gets wearing and very difficult. Like, right now my mother's very ill, so it's going to be even more difficult. . . . And I'll tell you, the few times that I have walked away, I get just an incredible feeling. When you've drawn the line and you're not doing this reevaluating, and you're not having any contact, and you're living a normal life, it's just incredible. It's a wonderful feeling. You know, it's just wonderful. You go out with friends. I mean, you don't think about it. It's just great. . . . But it's always constantly reevaluation. That's the most difficult thing.

ACCOUNTANT, *age thirty-five, daughter*

⤙

I'm responsible because I'm the closest person to her. So, anything that may happen is obviously my responsibility, not only on the basis of laws but also only the moral aspect. I mean, she is my mom. She raised me up all by herself. And if you look at me now, I'm all in good health. And I owe all the thanks to her and nobody else. I can be very sure of that. . . . There is a special sense of obligation that children have for their parents in Italy. So, on one hand . . . I really feel the responsibility. I mean, it's not something that I've been given. It's something that I take. On the other hand, my mom really cuts my wings. I mean, when she gets ill, I have to take care of her. I cannot do certain things. For example, I know that if I were to move here [United States], I would have a better job here and it would be a new chapter, a good opportunity for my life. And, I don't really know if I can take her here with me. So, I'm debating. In my heart, I know that my mom is first and before anything. But after all, is it first before my [own] life? . . . So, sometimes it's very hard. I go through various kinds of moods in a very short range of time. One day, I feel that she raised me and this is the least I can do. On the other hand, I say, "What about me? Who cares about me? What did I do to deserve this?" I think it's very sad. . . . So, anyway, it's a problem and I don't have an answer for it.

SALESMAN, *age thirty, son*

The choice of caregivers can, of course, be as stark as staying or leaving. One woman, caring for a sick daughter, has not been in touch with her mentally ill mother for nearly fifteen years. Yet another interview centered on a young man's painful decision to finally leave his wife. However, the more usual concerns of the interviewees is how constantly to shuttle between distance and closeness in their efforts to provide ongoing support. The remainder of this chapter details the factors caregivers take into account as they try to solve the most vexing caregiving equation—calculating the appropriate levels of involvement necessary to help another in trouble without jeopardizing their own life, liberty, and pursuit of happiness.

Caregiving in Context

Human troubles are often characterized by moments of epiphany or revelation when, after long periods experienced as utter chaos and confusion, the nature of the problem suddenly *seems* clear.[10] In the case of illness, one such moment is receiving a diagnosis. Of course, a person's behaviors are sometimes so beyond the norms of civility and acceptability that the label *mental illness* is quickly attached to them. Flips into psychotic mania, attempts at suicide, or having robust hallucinations rarely go unnoticed or are passed off as being within the bounds of normalcy. Still, large numbers of people who are eventually deemed mentally ill go for months, even years, without an "official" diagnosis. Family members, therefore, sometimes equally go for months or years feeling anger, fear, confusion, and concern about a loved one's oppressive behaviors without being able to name them as illness. The point at which a person's troublesome behavior is transformed into a disease, via the pronouncements of medical experts, is typically a moment of epiphany for caregivers (and sometimes for patients). Such an epiphany is, however, only the beginning of an ongoing interpretive process aimed at establishing comfortable caregiving boundaries.

Hoping and Learning

It is difficult to overestimate the power of receiving a medical diagnosis. Since a diagnosis of mental illness remains deeply stigmatizing, it is not surprising that "patients" often reject it. Sometimes family members are similarly shocked by the mental illness diagnosis and their first impulse is also to reject it. One woman told me that "when I heard those words [mental illness] from a doctor, it scared the life out of me." When the doctor explained "You have a serious problem on your hands. This boy is absolutely manic-depressive, if not schizophrenic," her response was to think "Oh my, don't say that. . . . It's just emotion. He needs to talk to a counselor." Another mother confessed that she was "scared by everything that was happening. I didn't know what was going on with my son. My son wouldn't even talk to me. He was out of his mind. . . . You know, [I was thinking] things like is he going to be in this hospital for the rest of his life?" For most family members, though, a diagnosis clarifies a history of problems and generates hope that a deeply disruptive family member will finally be "cured."

> I loved getting the diagnosis. That was the best day of my life.
>
> PHYSICAL THERAPIST, *age forty-nine, mother*

~

> I'll tell you one of the best days of my life was when I got a phone call from the hospital telling me what they decided was wrong with him [husband] and they couldn't understand why I was so excited or happy.
>
> DAY CARE ATTENDANT, *age fifty-five, wife*

~

> Well, before she was diagnosed as being bipolar, I was seriously thinking about getting a divorce because she was just so argumentative. You know, after she was diagnosed *it was something.* It was not a character or a personality issue. . . . It was something that . . .

she had no obvious control over and could be treated with medication. That put a different light on it.

ELECTRONICS DESIGNER, *age sixty, husband*

↩

After he [brother] was diagnosed, they [doctors] seemed to have
hope. They thought he'd come off of meds and now it's to the point
he's going to be on meds for the rest of his life. I don't know if they
have actually said that but it is obvious. . . . The doctors and everyone
[initially] gave us that optimism.

STUDENT, *age seventeen, sister*

Once it becomes clear that the problem is mental illness—usually after a dramatic crisis—family members often go through a
period of actively learning about it. This may involve conversations
with medical people and sometimes extensive reading. This learning process is typically accompanied by heroic efforts to save or
cure the sick person. Heroic measures are more easily undertaken
at the outset of a catastrophic illness because sympathy margins remain wide and caregivers often believe that once an emotionally ill
person realizes how much he or she is cared about, they will get
better. Heroic measures also display strong commitment, something that individuals are expected to show when someone close is
in a crisis. At this point in a family member's illness career the caregiving role is normally embraced fully, enthusiastically, and optimistically. In effect, there is no constructed boundary between the
ill person and family member during the early stages of what is
now openly a "caring" role. If there has been any change, it is that
boundaries between well and sick family members become even
more porous than previously.

Several of his sisters had said to me, "Don't feel you have to stick
around for him because you feel sorry for him." But it never occurred to me [to leave]. I felt that I ought to help him get through

it. I always believed he could get through it, although there were times right in the middle of it when I thought, "My God."

CUSTOMER SERVICE REPRESENTATIVE, *age thirty-five, wife*

↬

I felt that if I worked hard enough and fast enough I could make her [daughter] better. Anything [the doctors] suggested I jumped on with great enthusiasm.

NURSE, *age fifty, mother*

↬

The hardest [thing] probably for me is realizing that I can't be wonder woman. I can't do it all. I came up here with this idea that I was going to go to classes for two years and then write a dissertation in a year and be out of here. . . . But . . . after his first hospitalization up here, obviously that was not going to happen. But . . . it still did not hit me. Nothing, none of this really hit home until probably this past year when he was so sick that they finally did ECT on him. . . . And what hit home to me with that was . . . okay, he is a pretty sick guy. So that made me say, "Am I going to run full force [in all areas of my life] and maybe lose him . . . or am I going to slow down myself a little bit and be able to accommodate some of his needs that I can accommodate?"

GRADUATE STUDENT, *age twenty-eight, wife*

Such efforts might continue for some time, even years, but with growing doubts about their efficacy. Unfortunately, in virtually every interview, respondents eventually had to come to the reluctant conclusion that initial hopes for a solution to the problem were an illusion. Those who thought the right combination of love and care, medication, and counseling would heal a sick spouse, child, sibling, or parent slowly came to the recognition that the problem was far more complex than they initially imagined. The imagery that an episode of mental illness could be fixed in the way doctors might help a broken bone to mend gave way to a consciousness of mental illness as a permanent condition. Unlike receiving a diagnosis, the recognition of mental illness' permanence seeps into caregivers' consciousness over time. Still, there must be a moment somewhere along the line when a caregiver finally acknowledges the idea that the problem is unlikely ever fully to disappear. That moment no doubt also constitutes an epiphany, albeit a negative one, that sets in motion a wholly new view of their relationship with the ill person in their lives.

While every respondent grappled with the concept of permanence, Angela, a forty-six-year-old woman whose life is bounded by a daughter, a sister, and mother with mental illness, as well as another child with cerebral palsy, summed up with great precision the changes in consciousness generated by having to admit that a mental illness may never go away. The matter of permanence came up in our conversation as we were talking about feelings of chronic loss and sorrow generated by her children's illnesses. Here, in some detail, is what she said:

> I guess I didn't feel her loss that much until after she [sister] tried to commit suicide. I mean I didn't feel like it would be permanent. ... You know, she did have these periods of getting better and so I didn't feel it as permanent. ... I always thought that maybe she would get better or she'd go to a different doctor. ... I still didn't see it as permanent. It was later.

> *So, are you saying that the loss becomes more profound at the moment of recognition of permanence?*

> Oh definitely, for her [mother] and for my daughter. That [recognition] is just devastating. Well, if it is not permanent it is like having a cold or something. I mean you go through this period and the person is really unhappy. ... [For example], you go through labor and you have a child. They'll be an end to it. And at the end, you know, all of your efforts and suffering will have been for something, you feel. But when you finally realize that there is no end, then you

have a whole different mind-set so you have to change. . . . First of all, a lot of your sympathy and support will dry up because people are going to get sick of doing that [caretaking]. . . . So you'll be out there alone, sort of trekking along, trying to support them because . . . whatever happens to that person, no matter how bad they get, whatever happens, you are not going to desert them. That is how I feel with my . . . mother and my daughter. . . . I will try to offer some level of support and be there for them.

So if it is permanent, then my whole life has changed and I have to offer this kind of support that I don't really want to offer, but I feel like I have to. And I wouldn't feel like a decent person if I didn't. . . . You know, my mother may die in a few years. My sister may be alive for all of my life, but she has her husband. . . . But with all of them, it is to some extent that you feel like that. But with my daughter I felt it most profoundly. When it's not permanent you can withstand almost anything. When it's permanent, its completely different.

INSURANCE ADMINISTRATOR, *age forty-six, daughter/sister*

Revising Expectations

Erik Erikson has written that it is the capacity for hope that most significantly distinguishes human beings from other animals.[11] Indeed, as the writings of Bruno Bettelheim[12] and Viktor Frankl[13] on the holocaust so powerfully illustrate, human beings are remarkably able to sustain hope in even the most horrific circumstances imaginable. We should not be surprised, therefore, that even when the recognition of mental illness's permanence settles into their consciousness and seriously erodes the belief that a resolution of the problem is possible, respondents rarely lose hope altogether. At the point in our conversation when we discuss the chronic nature of mental illness and the likelihood that it will be a lifelong problem, caregivers sometimes follow their realistic assessment of things with the nearly apologetic statement, "But I still can't help but to feel hope." In the self-help group at McLean's, a repeating theme of the talk, often invoked after someone has detailed a particularly difficult situation, is the observation that the medications for mental illness are getting better all the time and that medical science might even one day solve the problem. Nevertheless, nearly everyone interviewed described how they felt obliged to ratchet down their expectations for the person in their care.

> I gave up the future .... She is really lost to us as the kid that we knew and the relationship that we had. This is gone. We are grieving the final loss. And they [doctors] said to me, "She might come back." And I said, "I can't do that. I have to grieve that she is totally gone and that she's not coming back in any sense that we knew her." Not that we will never see her again, but that she is not coming back in any sense that we knew her. ... Anything that I get from this point forward is a gift and not a disappointment. ... Oh, I sob my guts out. But I'm not sorry for me. I mean, once in a while I say, "This sucks. This is awful. Why do I feel so terrible?" But that's like really rare. I lost this kid. I lost the last piece of this kid. I sob for my loss. I don't sob for me. Does that make sense to you?
>
> PHYSICAL THERAPIST, *age forty-nine, mother*

> You have to realize that the person is not going to be what you want them to be or not going to have the life you would like for them.
>
> ACCOUNTANT, *age thirty-five, daughter*

Caregivers also ratchet down expectations for their own lives.

> We almost had to put our life on hold. I find we're five years behind all of our friends. We just bought a house. Most of our friends bought a house when they were in their late twenties. And ... last March, about kids, I finally got up the guts, and said "Okay, I want to start talking about kids. It's really on my mind. It's bothering me. All of our friends have kids. All of our friends are now on their second kid by this point. And ... it's hitting me." Up until then, it hadn't even hit me. And so we talked about it. And, you know, I

said to Tom, "I'm not talking about getting pregnant tomorrow. I just want you to know this is what's going through my mind." The kids thing came up again around Christmas time . . . and we said we'll talk about it in a little bit. And then, when Tom went through this depression a couple of weeks ago, I thought to myself, "My God, what would happen if I had a child? All this energy for years I've put into Tom, I'm not going to have anymore." So, that's a big case scenario. Everything I do I have to think about how's this going to affect Tom. . . . So, I mean, we're at the point now where we still put off the decision. God help me when I turn forty [*laughing*], but we still have a couple more years.

CUSTOMER SERVICE REPRESENTATIVE, *age thirty-five, wife*

In order not to leave you with the mistaken impression that all caregivers eventually feel utterly fatalistic about the future, I should say that some also describe feelings of efficacy and progress in their efforts to help. Although admitting that it is still difficult for them to figure out exactly what they might realistically expect for their son's future, Eileen and Bill are optimistic. From the time Ray suffered a severe psychotic episode, the trajectory of his illness has been toward greater health. He has returned to school and recently began a new job. Eileen observed that "he's thinking really clearly and pacing himself and monitoring himself. I think most of our work with him is over really." And Bill added, "I guess one of the things we've learned is . . . about taking time. These things do not just flip into the next phase just like that. It just keeps evolving [in a positive direction]. . . . Progress is being made and . . . we've learned stuff and Ray has learned stuff and we have a relationship with the doctor and we have some sense of what to do and what not to do."

Even among those who report progress, the dominant theme of the interviews is an increasing recognition that, despite their best efforts at caretaking, the problem will remain. At a point, everyone also realizes that they truly cannot control the course of another's mental illness and must surrender to that reality. Perceiving their inability to control things is exceedingly important because once that becomes a caretaker's prevailing view, it calls forth renewed efforts to recast the boundaries of obligation. The realization that intractable illness thwarts their earlier goal of control is an "identity turning point" in the careers of caregivers.[14] Now, they feel more disposed to accept the inevitability of the problem, to define it more thoroughly in disease terms, and, consequently, to feel less responsible for the unfortunate consequences of their family member's illness.

> I was tired. I was fed up. I was really angry at her. . . . I was furious at her for two months. . . . One of the things that I kept saying was, "I think what I'm going through is the last stage of acceptance." . . . I mean, part of it was [that] in order to accept her illness I had to let go of my responsibility. . . . My feeling, where I sit right now is that . . . I have absolutely no control over her. She can go off her medication. She can totally, excuse me, fuck up her life and I have no control over that. I can't stop it. . . . I think that is the acceptance I got to last December.
>
> PHYSICAL THERAPIST, *age forty-nine, mother*

↫

> And by that point he had pulled away from everybody. He wouldn't see anybody. So I mean, it was just a train heading [toward a crash]. There was nothing I could do. . . . Every time I thought I was helping, it was making things worse. So, I guess I must have at some point just sat back and said, "I'm doing all I can and if something else happens, I know I've done my best."
>
> CUSTOMER SERVICE REPRESENTATIVE, *age thirty-five, wife*

↫

> I would love to be able to state what Diane's life is going to be, but I have no control over it.
>
> HOMEMAKER, *age seventy-two, mother*

A caregiver's dual recognition that (1) mental illness is unlikely ever to be resolved and (2) that they cannot control it, leads to a fundamental reassessment of their felt obligations. At this juncture in their relationship with an ill family member, caregivers begin to ask themselves with increasing frequency the question "What are my spouse's (or my child's, my sibling's, my parent's) obligations to care for themselves?" Once that question seriously arises in their consciousness, wholly new perceptions and emotions about their role in an ill person's life become possible.

Assessing Responsibility

In his comprehensive history of Darwinian thought, Carl Degler points out that biological explanations of human nature dominated America's thinking at the turn of the century, but then fell into disfavor for decades.[15] Within the last ten to fifteen years, biological explanations of human behavior have made a big comeback. The prevailing wisdom in American psychiatry seems to be that affective disorders are brain diseases. Advocate groups such as NAMI (National Alliance for the Mentally Ill) fully embrace the view that people suffering from depression, manic-depression, and schizophrenia have "broken brains," in effect. Although members of the MDDA support group occasionally express some reservations about the biological basis for mental illness, versions of biological determinism dominate the talk when questions of cause arise.[16] Likewise, nearly everyone interviewed for this book, although willing to speculate about the social or situational factors that might kick off an illness episode, ultimately saw their loved one's problem as a product of bad brain chemistry.

My purpose here certainly is not to unravel how nature and nurture might combine in the case of mental illness. Whatever might be the cause(s) of mental illness, I understand the appeal of biological explanations, both for caregivers and those afflicted. If the problem is essentially biological, caregivers and their loved ones are largely absolved from responsibility—caregivers from the responsibility of somehow having caused a family member's anguish and ill persons from responsibility for their unacceptable behavior.

Biological explanations, by understanding mental illness as somehow rooted in neurotransmitters gone awry, significantly insulate caregivers and patients from moral blame. However, despite generally embracing biological explanations, caregivers who routinely deal with a family member's difficult, hurtful, and unreasonable behaviors inevitably navigate a difficult explanatory course between determinism and personal responsibility. It is a caregiving paradox that while speaking the language of biological determinism, caregivers still invoke personal responsibility as a criterion for assessing the extent of their obligations.

Once again, the case of mental illness raises distinctive puzzles for caregivers. I have already discussed how perceptions of permanence and an inability to control the ill person's behavior shape feelings of duty and responsibility over time. To these socially rooted caregiving contingencies let me now add another—the relative willingness of patients to comply with medical treatment. Because of the stigma attached to the mental illness label, the debilitating side effects of powerful psychotropic medications, and often the inability of mentally ill people to appreciate how strange their behaviors seem to others, many ill family members simply deny that they are sick and, thus, refuse any form of treatment.

In those families where an ill person does not comply with medical treatment, the reservoir of caregiving sympathy quickly evaporates. Among support group members, conversations often center on strategies for getting family members to accept that they have a disease and to comply with medical protocols. Whether or not their ill spouse, child, parent, or sibling undergoes therapeutic treatments, everyone interviewed agreed that they must bear significant responsibility for getting well. Exhibiting such responsibility becomes, at a certain point, the *sine qua non* of their willingness to continue as caregivers. Rachel, who has been caring for two siblings, captures sentiments expressed repeatedly in the interviews:

> It is a complicated thing with mental illness because, on the one
> hand, if you buy the idea that people really do have . . . a brain

disorder, [that] there's something wrong with the serotonin levels or something in [their] head, well then you really can't hold people . . . responsible for their behavior. . . . But it's also got to be pretty hard to hear from somebody who is saying, "[There is] nothing I can do. I am just sick and that is it." . . . I mean, it is hard to hear that and I guess the difference between my brother and sister is that when he first got sick, he pretty much almost immediately assumed a major part of the responsibility for his illness. I mean, he has worked. He has gone to school. He has read books. He has gone to support groups. He has had regular medical appointments. For the most part he has been compliant with medicine for the better portion of the time he has been sick. He has listened to people [and] gotten advice. I mean, he is not perfect at dealing with it, but that [compliance] really is what has to happen. I would say the same thing about my sister's illness or my mother's alcoholism. The sin isn't in being sick. The real sin is people who simply don't accept [their illness] and [don't] get the help that they need so that they can at least attempt to help themselves. . . . Until they get to the point of helping themselves, you know, the best psychiatrists in the world and pills are just no magic potion because there is a lot of work that has to be done. And you know, I suppose some people just say, "It's too much work. I am not going to bother to get better. It's too painful." And I think that is where my sister is at. She just sees it as too daunting a job. Better to be sick than [to] crack away at some of the things that have shaped her whole life—her identity of depression. I mean, that is how she identifies herself—with depression and a depressed life; not being able to go anywhere and not having any goals or aspirations.

TECHNOLOGY LICENSER, *age thirty-three, sister*

Research exploring the distribution of empathy suggests that, based on principles of distributive justice, we most thoroughly empathize with those whom we consider hardworking.[17] In a society bounded by a history of Protestant ethic ideologies and a cultural ethos of individualistic achievement, empathy is especially accorded those who show a willingness to "pull themselves up by their boot-

straps." Welfare debates in the United States center on identification of the "truly disadvantaged" and the "deserving needy."[18] Increasingly, both federal and state governments seem disposed to
provide welfare only to those who are viewed as willing to help
themselves. Similarly, caregivers nearly always came to feel that they
should continue to extend themselves only if their family member
seemed to be making a good faith effort to help themselves.

> Until it got down to the essence of him having to be responsible for
> his own actions [our marriage was in trouble]. . . . Now I feel that
> it's a much more healthy [situation] . . . because he really is respond-
> ing. . . . Joe is willing to work hard at this [staying well]. . . . I keep
> saying to him, "You have only one soul to save and that's your own."
> If you are saving your soul you won't be a burden to anyone
> else. . . . I am very fortunate that he is so motivated, that he wants
> to figure this out. He wants to have a good life.
>
> NURSE, *age fifty, wife*

⤶

> I feel that even if they have a mental illness, there are responsibilities
> that go along with the mental illness. . . . You see your doctor when
> you're supposed to. You take your medication as you're supposed
> to. You live as healthy a lifestyle that you can. If it means that there
> are people in your life that contribute to your mental illness, then
> you avoid those people. You absolutely have some control over your
> own mental illness. . . . With mental illness, yes, it's something that's
> going on in the body that you don't have any control over. But if it
> means you avoid alcohol to keep it controlled, then you don't drink.
> If it means you need to walk a half-hour every day to get the sero-
> tonin levels up, then you walk that half-hour every day. Take
> charge!!! Don't think that it's somebody else's responsibilities.
>
> RETIRED SECRETARY, *age fifty-eight, mother*

The interpretive problem of deciding just how strenuously to
draw caregiving boundaries is additionally complicated by the perceived difficulty in determining whether someone's troublesome be-

haviors truly arise from that person's mental illness. As the previous comments indicate, caregivers invariably wonder whether a mentally ill person can, in fact, exercise control over many of their problematic behaviors. Consequently, caregivers routinely face the dilemma of deciding whether to hold the *person* or the *disease* responsible for objectionable behaviors. Although those sick with physical illnesses may sometimes be accused of abusing the "sick role," caregivers ordinarily feel able to determine the authenticity of their complaints and the propriety of their inability to fulfill social obligations.[19] The matter is more opaque in the case of mental illness. As a result, respondents in this study often described how caregiving boundaries were frayed by the suspicion that the ill person in their life sometimes manipulates them.

> Well, I think . . . that with someone who has mental illness . . . there is definitely a component of [it] that they have some control over. I don't think that our understanding of mental illness is such that we believe that the person has no control over this. . . . If she [mother] had cancer [instead of mental illness] and she was bedridden, you can kind of understand that. Like her body [doesn't work], you know. And everyone else is validating her. Everyone else around her, like the doctors, are validating the fact that she is sick. She really can't get out of bed. You know, that is what she needs. You know? She needs this treatment. [But] when everyone else around you is saying to you, "It's in her head," and you are trying to do [things] for her and she is not . . . responding to you, you are thinking to yourself, "She could be trying to do more."
>
> RESEARCH ASSISTANT, *age twenty-three, daughter*

∽

> I also got angry because I really view a lot of it as being manipulative and the older I got, the angrier I got at him [father] because I could see that he could control it when he wanted to. . . . When I was growing up he could control it around who he wanted to. Maybe there were a couple of isolated incidents where he really couldn't,

but for the majority of it he would switch like that [*snaps fingers*] when somebody else came around. . . . There was a tremendous amount of control there that he was not exerting and so I got angry because he would manipulate. He would manipulate in the sense that he would want everybody's pity, but he wouldn't do anything anybody suggested.

LAWYER, *age thirty-three, daughter*

↜

I think the illness breeds a certain form of manipulation. Some of it is that you know the person is manipulating you and some of it is, you know, they really aren't well and this is their survival skill.

TECHNOLOGY LICENSER, *age thirty-three, sister*

Chapter 3 will deal with the incredibly strong, frequently negative, and nearly always ambivalent emotions that interviewees feel toward a mentally disabled family member. The emotions surrounding caregiving become especially complicated when people have feelings that they consider illegitimate. That is, the problems of managing emotions are compounded when people feel a second order of emotions, emotions about their emotions. The interviews are replete with expressions of embarrassment, shame, and guilt for feeling anger, resentment, or even hate toward a person you are supposed to love.

A growing body of literature on the sociology of emotions centers on the idea that we do not simply feel emotions; we also create, intensify, suppress, and transform them.[20] One relevant question to ask, therefore, is "How do people deal with emotions when culturally given 'feeling rules' are not well-developed?"[21] I can say with clarity right now that, in the case of mental illness, feelings about caregiving evolve to the point where individuals are forced to entertain these questions: "What are the circumstances under which I would have to leave? What are my limits as a caregiver?" The final data section of this chapter focuses on their answers.

Preserving Oneself

There is a methodological bias in the sample of people assembled for this study. Because many of them were recruited from a "Family and Friends" self-help group, they are people who are sufficiently invested in the caregiving role to participate weekly at the meetings. This is, therefore, primarily a study of how people who have elected to stay in a caregiving relationship bear responsibility. My generalizations cannot extend to those who have given up and exited from the lives of mentally ill relatives. However, several respondents certainly have a perspective on family members who either are not doing their fair share of caregiving or have left altogether. One of my interviews was with the eldest daughter in a large family who was faced with virtually the sole responsibility of caring for her schizophrenic mother. Ordinarily, Joanna simply assumed that it was her duty to be The Caregiver, saying at one point, "I was born with the obligation." However, feelings of resentment toward family members who were literally "hiding out" from her mother (by having unlisted telephone numbers and not revealing their home addresses) surfaced on the occasion of a funeral. Here's the scene Joanna described:

> Her brothers and sisters, yes, they're hiding out. She does have contact with one sister. This sister has a lot of problems too. It's not a good situation for them to be together. But yes. . . . I'm really angry at the fact that they did that. Absolutely. I still can't comprehend how somebody could do that. I really haven't given it much thought until I went to my grandmother's funeral back in January. And I realized that everybody was so uncomfortable, and everybody was so concerned with my mother's being there, and the fact that I brought her. I realized that, you know, "She's your sister as much as she's my mother, and she's sick." And they were looking at me like, "Can't you take her somewhere or do something with her?" And I'm thinking, "You know, you're not here [for her] now. You should have been there years ago, too." I try to forget about it, because

confronting them about it or expressing how I feel about it just doesn't seem to have achieved anything. But I absolutely had some resentment for that toward her siblings and her parents.

ACCOUNTANT, age thirty-five, daughter

Interestingly, when people talk about family members who have opted out of any caregiving, they rarely express rancor toward them. While upset by their own caregiving burden, they seem to understand the motives of those who have left. Their understanding, even compassion, for relatives who do not help them with an ill family member is possible in a culture that deifies personal freedom and the obligation of individuals to achieve *self*-fulfillment. Indeed, as one of my graduate students from Thailand periodically reminds me, the obligation issues that so confound the people interviewed for this study do not exist in her country. She reports that the question "Shall I subordinate my own needs and desires to the task of caring for a sick spouse, child, parent, or sibling?" cannot even arise in the consciousness of a Thai family member. There simply is no competing expectation to the cultural demand that one be a devoted caregiver.

Although the sociological analysis of individualism extends to the origins of the discipline, the conversation about its significance in understanding American character and social structure was reinvigorated through the writings of Robert Bellah and his colleagues. *Habits of the Heart* details how the ethic of individualism in the United States fosters self-absorption and guarantees a collective sense of strangeness, isolation, and loneliness.[22] At one point, the authors discuss the deep ambivalence Americans have about freedom and attachment. The dilemma posed by the need both for attachment and freedom is beautifully captured in Bellah's analysis of romantic love in America. On the one side, Americans believe deeply in romantic love as a necessary requirement for self-satisfaction. At the same time, love and marriage, which are based on the free giving of self to another, pose the problem that in sharing too completely with another one might lose oneself. The difficulties that Americans have in maintaining intimate relationships stem in part from the uneasy balance between sharing and being separate. The argument is put this way:

> Love, then, creates a dilemma for Americans. In some ways, love is the quintessential experience of individuality and freedom. At the same time, it offers intimacy, mutuality, and sharing. In the ideal love relationship, these two aspects of love are perfectly joined—love is both absolutely free and completely shared. Such moments of perfect harmony among free individuals are rare, however. The sharing and commitment in a love relationship can seem, for some, to swallow up the individual, making her (more often than him) lose sight of her own interests, opinions, and desires. . . . Losing a sense of one's self may also lead to being exploited, or even abandoned, by the person one loves.[23]

Certainly, as the quotes throughout this chapter suggest, the task of caregiving is often deeply connected with the privilege of loving. That being so, the ambivalence felt by caregivers as they search for the proper balance of attachment and separation arises from precisely the same cultural confusions that compromise our capacity to love. My data affirm Bellah's theoretical observations that the fear of losing oneself is what ultimately motivates people to leave relationships that threaten to engulf them. When asked what might persuade them to exit from their caregiving situation, most of the respondents first declared that they were unlikely ever to back away completely from their caring obligations. When pressed further, though, they commonly articulated three fundamental criteria that might require exiting—the realization that their efforts to care are ineffective, feeling that their own health is seriously jeopardized by caring, and believing that their self or identity is in danger of obliteration because of their relationship with a mentally ill person.

> I know . . . my limit is reached [when] all I think about is . . . getting her [mother] in the car and driving off a cliff because I can't stand

to be with her and I feel she can't do this to people any more. . . . In a way my identity disappeared because I was just sucked into that blackness and weirdness. . . . For me, this is my parent and I felt like she was destroying me and I hated her for that. But then I thought this is my mother and she loves me . . . I have very little sympathy, which is sort of cruel of me.

INSURANCE ADMINISTRATOR, *age forty-six, daughter/sister*

↜

I reach some limit in terms of support. . . . I had stood by him through a number of drunk episodes and situations where he was suicidally depressed. . . . I've seen him fuck up his relationships over and over again, and I was there for him. . . . I did not cut this person off easily. But I reach the point with my own mental health [where] I could not take his abusiveness anymore. I just felt like I had to take care of myself and I couldn't [help him] anymore.

RESEARCH PROFESSOR, *age forty-seven, sister*

↜

The breaking point that I am referring to is where I just . . . am not going anywhere with this and I think that I am not going to be able to help her, and the marriage is probably going down the drain. . . . I have tried every venue to help my wife and I am not helping her and at the same time I am destroying myself.

SHOP MANAGER, *age twenty-six, husband*

↜

In the last year . . . either I reached my saturation point or I realized how detrimental it was to my personal health. . . . [My therapist] really helped put it in perspective and we sat down for forty minutes and we drew out a little grid and I think that is when he basically pinpointed it. He goes, "You can't do any more than you are doing and at some point you have to just walk away and say 'I can't do it.'"

LAWYER, *age thirty-three, daughter*

The data and analysis presented in this chapter, aside from complementing existing quantitative studies on caregiving, suggest that different illnesses generate distinctive caregiving contingencies. I have maintained that mental illness poses its own unique interpretive dilemmas for caregivers. With greater frequency than for most physical illnesses, mentally ill persons will reject medical diagnoses, will refuse to participate in efforts to become well, will be angry and hostile toward caregivers, and will be unable to express gratitude for the care they receive. Because these dimensions of mental illness may not be wholly apparent at the outset of caregiving efforts, perspectives on caring shift over time. Initial definitions of appropriate responsibility boundaries prove inadequate as a caregiver's consciousness about a family member's mental illness evolves.

Although I am hesitant to describe caregivers' perspectival shifts in terms of predictable stages, I have identified four interpretive "junctures" in an individual's efforts to care for a mentally ill family member. Early in a patient's illness career, caregiving boundaries are expansively drawn and extensive efforts are often made to "cure" an afflicted person's illness. At some point, caregivers realize that while there may be periods of remission, mental illness is likely to be a lifelong condition. This causes caregivers to revise life expectations both for themselves and the ill person in their care. An understanding that the problem may be permanent, along with an eventual awareness of their inability to control the ill person's behaviors, moves caregivers to yet again reassess their responsibilities. In particular, they gauge their own obligation by the ill person's willingness to comply with medical treatment. Such thinking about joint responsibility often requires delicately balancing biological views of mental illness's cause with ideologies of personal responsibility. Finally, caregivers may, at some point, discontinue care. Such a decision is related to the unhappy realization that nothing they try is effective in ameliorating the problem and that continued caring will fundamentally undermine their own health and the integrity of their identity.

Throughout I have avoided such descriptors as "the caregiving role" or "the caregiving burden."[24] Certainly, the words of respondents imply the existence of broadly held cultural scripts about the obligation to care. However, the notion of a singular caregiving role implies a consistency and uniformity of experience that does not adequately address the contextual factors that shape caregiving. The notion of a caregiving role does not sufficiently attend to how a caregiver's phenomenology shifts as clarity about the character of mental illness emerges over time. Put in slightly different terms, the interview materials highlight the dialectical, processual, and emergent relationship between sufferers of any illness and those who care for them. The data illustrate that the moral boundaries of caregiving are constantly "under construction," dependent as they are on the meanings generated through the ongoing interactions of caregivers and patients.

Arthur Frank writes, "Caregivers are the other halves of illness experiences. The care they give begins by doing things for ill persons, but turns into sharing the life they lead."[25] And later, "Eventually a balance must be worked out between what the ill person needs and what the caregivers are able to provide."[26] This chapter has been directed at learning how the lives of caregivers and mentally ill family members become intertwined and how caregivers try to sustain workable levels of responsibility. A more thorough account of how obligation boundaries are created must consider the "social locations" of caregivers—their status within the family. Chapters 4 will examine how this social dimension affects the willingness of individuals to care.

A more immediate task, though, is suggested by comments of those who have spoken in this chapter. Caregiving arouses profound and complicated emotions. We ought to expect that as feelings of obligation shift over the natural history of an illness career, so also will the dominant emotions felt by family caregivers. Chapter 3 fills out the general picture I have begun to create by detailing how caregivers manage the powerful emotions that accompany meeting moral obligations.

THREE

Managing Emotions

You hate her illness, but you don't hate her. And I hate
what she has done to us and the hell that she has put
us through. . . . I don't think that I hate her. . . . I think
that it's more hating the illness. . . . I try to tell myself
that it's not her. . . . It's not "I hate *you*." It's "I hate
what you have done. I hate what you are doing."

ACCOUNTANT, *age thirty-five, daughter*

Although sociologists have always understood feelings of obligation, responsibility, and duty to be the moral cornerstones of society, little attention has been given to the ways such feelings are
evoked, interpreted, managed, and acted on in everyday life. Candace Clark has observed that while "Sociologists often use the language of reciprocity and exchange to explain the give-and-take of
everyday interaction . . . [they] rarely ask why people feel they owe
something to others, what the 'ligament' is that connects people,
or what the feeling of owing or obligation consists of."[1] This chapter examines the intense emotions that surround efforts to honor a
commitment to care for a family member with a major mental illness. My goal is to explain the kinds of emotions that arise as family members engage in ongoing interpretations of what they owe a
spouse, child, parent, brother, or sister in desperate emotional
trouble.

It is not surprising that severe illness makes particularly ex-
hausting emotional demands on healthy family members. In one
survey, 48.1 percent of the sample named the serious illness, suicide,
or death of a loved one as generating emotions other than what

respondents thought they "ought" to feel.[2] As difficult as it is to manage emotions in caring for a physically ill person, efforts to negotiate appropriate emotions are still more arduous in dealing with a mentally ill person. Since shared moods and feelings are necessary for the maintenance of social life, mentally ill people especially disrupt family life because they suffer from an "affective" disorder. The diagnoses of depression or manic-depression are partly defined by a person's inability to feel "correct" emotions.[3]

While their sickness might dramatically disrupt the logistical routines of everyday family life, physically ill people are ordinarily deeply invested in getting well and returning to their presickness social roles. In contrast, mentally ill persons, virtually by definition, cannot abide by the usual rules of social settings and behave in socially unacceptable ways. Sometimes they deny that they are ill, and frequently treat their caregivers with hostility instead of gratitude. Further, if ordinary social interaction requires the ability of persons to see the world from each other's perspectives, efforts at meaningful communication with the mentally ill are typically short-circuited. After all, they have been identified as mentally ill because they have feelings and thoughts that are incomprehensible to "healthy" persons. In this way, mentally ill people threaten both the concrete routines of daily life and, more significantly, the implicit symbolic order on which such routines are premised. Their behaviors are especially disturbing because they upset the most sacred of all social things—the coherence of everyday life.

With its emphasis on how caregivers negotiate their feelings, this chapter contributes to the emerging study of the "sociology of emotions."[4] Caring for emotionally ill people highlights the "links between cultural ideas, structural arrangements and . . . the way we wish we felt, the way we try to feel, the way we feel, the way we show what we feel, and the way we pay attention to, label, and make sense of what we feel."[5] The problematic character of the emotions generated by mental illness makes it a strategically useful case for advancing our understanding of what Arlie Russell Hochschild has called "emotion work."[6] Because breaches of social order generate exceptionally strong negative emotions, the case of mental illness allows us to examine how caregivers reconcile love for a family member with such emotions as fear, bewilderment, frustration, resentment, anger, and even hate.[7]

As in the last chapter, I begin here with the assumption that the caregiving experience must be looked at as a process. In their earlier and groundbreaking research, Barney Glaser and Anselm Strauss demonstrated that illnesses follow clear and predictable social trajectories.[8] In my own work[9] on depression, I argue that people afflicted with mental illness follow a discernible "career" path characterized by critical "turning points in identity."[10] To the extent that there are predictable moments in the unfolding of a family member's illness, there is a parallel caregiving career. In Chapter 2, I showed that caregivers' views of their obligations change over time. In this chapter, I will detail the corresponding shifts in the emotions they feel about giving care.

By considering the evolution of caregivers' emotions, I am moving beyond studies that link emotions only to particular incidences, momentary encounters, or discrete events. Hochschild has noted that her own well-received work, *The Managed Heart*, analyzed feeling rules and emotion management *only during troubling moments*.[11] This recognition has led her to call for studies that "ask by what principle . . . we manage our feelings over the course of a long string of moments; how . . . we fit emotion management to a line of action through time."[12] In a similar vein, Steven Gordon says that "we need studies of how people . . . negotiate and bargain over a norm's exact context and situational applicability."[13] This chapter derives its conceptual energy by examining the relationship between obligations and emergent emotions. Consideration of how emotions systematically change over the joint caregiver/patient career illuminates how the emotions we feel at any moment in time may be rooted in a prior history of affect.

Although students of emotion have rarely looked at the interactional history of emotions, they have nevertheless provided a useful conceptual tool for doing so. Hochschild has proposed the idea of "framing rules"[14] as an aid for comprehending the linkage between ideologies and emotions. As an example, a woman who has embraced certain principles of feminism may feel differently about leaving her children in a day-care center than a woman who feels no affinity with feminist ideologies. The behavior of the two women is identical—leaving a child in the care of others—but their respective and different framing rules will yield different emotions. Although our later discussion does relate caregivers' emotions to the essentially ideological frame of mental illness as a brain disease, my use of the framing concept is politically neutral. I will show how each phase or turning point in the caregiver/patient career is characterized by a distinctive cognitive frame that shapes respondents' emotions.

In order not to simplify things too much, I should say that those interviewed felt a range and simultaneity of emotions throughout the course of their relationship with the ill person in their lives. In fact, part of the difficulty posed by mental illness is the sheer volume and volatility of the emotions experienced. Everyone with whom I spoke felt fear, confusion, hope, compassion, sympathy, love, frustration, sadness, grief, anger, resentment, and guilt. Equally clear, however, are the consistent changes in the relative significance and intensity of each of these emotions over time. You might think of the several emotions felt by respondents as constituting a shifting hierarchy of emotional salience. Thus, my analysis is directed toward documenting and accounting for the dominant emotions at each critical juncture of the common path shared by the caregivers in this study.

Paralleling Chapter 2, I look at the ebb and flow of emotions at four critical junctures in the caregiver/patient career. Prior to a firm medical diagnosis, respondents experience what I call *emotional anomie*.[15] They are grossly confused by the behaviors of a family member and quite simply don't know precisely what to feel. Anomie refers to the sheer bewilderment of a life that has quickly shifted from coherence and predictability to chaos and disorder. Eventually, a diagnosis of depression, manic-depression, or schizophrenia provides a medical frame that clarifies the circumstance of caregivers and provokes feelings of hope, compassion, and sympathy. At a certain point, initial optimism that their loved one's mental illness can be fixed gives way to a sense of its likely permanence. The frame of permanence, coupled with doubts about the ill person's inability to control objectionable behaviors, ushers in more negative feelings of anger, resentment, even hate. Some of the respondents eventually conclude that none of their efforts can successfully change things. Such a recognition leads them to an acceptance of the other's condition. Acceptance has the potential to liberate caregivers from the earlier burdensome belief that it is their duty to somehow solve the problem.

Experiencing Emotional Anomie

As sociologists have long observed, the decision that someone is suffering from mental illness is certainly as much a cultural and political decision as it is a purely medical one.[16] Parents of adolescents or young adults often found it particularly confusing to make sense of their children's extremely troubling behaviors since they were moving through a life stage normally associated with difficult and contrary behaviors. Several parents described long periods during which they were uncertain what to make of their children's behaviors or how to respond to them. Here are the reactions of some typical parents during this early stage in their child's illness:

> Well the lines are blurred. . . . But you know what mental illness is. . . . At least if you're psychotic, you know that. That is different from just rebelling and for four years Brad was sort of doing [that]. . . . But my horror was just the experience of knowing that your son is decompensating (*sic*). . . . You don't know whether he is on drugs or what is going on with this kid. You don't know what to do if he is. If he's on drugs, do you call the police? Do you call the doctor? Maybe he's not on drugs. Maybe this kid is just, you know, acting

[out]. I mean I never saw a real crazy person in my life. You hear of the crazy all the time, but I never saw anybody doing what he was doing and acting and saying the things he was saying. . . . [It's] massive chaos.

SECRETARY, *age fifty-three, mother*

↩

One of the hardest things for me before she was diagnosed was what was I doing wrong as a mother. . . . Back then it was just sort of this amorphous mess. All of a sudden she was someone [I didn't know]. She felt out of control to me. But I couldn't label the behaviors. There was no way that I could have said, "This belongs to an illness," because she hadn't been diagnosed. I had no understanding of that illness. . . . I mean, it took me two years to understand all that it meant to have a daughter who was mentally ill. I worked on coming to terms with that for two years.

GRADE SCHOOL TEACHER, *age forty-eight, mother*

Although adolescence might precipitate the greatest measure of confusion about whether to label a set of behaviors as mental illness, deciding whether to call someone mentally ill can pose dilemmas across the life span. The following are the comments of a young woman who tried to convey her guilt for doubting whether her mother was truly mentally ill. Her words also illustrate the extraordinary jumble of emotions we can feel when the causes of a loved one's demanding behaviors are unclear:

I am sitting there and I am second-guessing my mom. You know? And I am going to the doctors and a lot of the doctors are saying that it is [all] in her head. . . . The burning sensations and the fact that her jaw was bothering her too and we had to . . . process her food and stuff for her. And so I am sitting there and I have my mom who, you know, has taught me everything I know about morals and ethics and I am second-guessing her now, someone who I hold in so much respect. And I am second-guessing her. I am feeling bad

for second-guessing her when I am really wondering what is going
on and I am doubting her and it hurts to doubt your mom.... I
was just confused. I was totally confused and . . . I could never deal
with everything at once because there were just so many different
emotions, just because there was all of the doubt.

RESEARCH ASSISTANT, *age twenty-three, daughter*

The kind of pervasive confusion described thus far is, of course,
most likely in those instances in which a person's ability to function
unravels slowly and over a long period of time. However, mental
illness can strike with unimagined ferocity, ripping through a family
like a suddenly emerging tornado that allows no preparation. It hits
quickly and leaves utter devastation and confusion as its aftermath.
Time and again, I heard stories like that of the parents who received
a call from India that their son, spending a year abroad, had gone
mad. In absolute bewilderment they had to fly to India immediately
to prevent his incarceration. In other cases, telephone calls that
thoroughly changed the course of people's lives came from a child's
college roommates who could no longer cope with his bizarre behaviors or a girlfriend who was literally being held hostage in a
son's room.

In these and similar cases there is no question that something is
drastically wrong and that some sort of emotional disorder is involved. Stories of this kind invariably included a respondent's first
contact with doctors and hospitals, experiences that only exacerbated the trauma of mental illness's sudden, totally unanticipated
appearance. For example, consider further the plight of the parents
who had to retrieve their son from India. After a harrowing trip
back to the United States, during which their psychotic son tried
several times to escape from the plane, they finally got him into a
psychiatric hospital. His hospital admission, however, did little to
assuage their fears or clarify what precisely was wrong.

We were just scared. . . . We had this collection of doctors and social
workers all sort of staring at us because we were trying to explain

what had happened, but nobody was really interested in what we had to say . . . because we were not the patient. . . . From the nurse's point of view, we were being blamed. . . . "Why did you let this person . . . go run around the streets? He should be hospitalized." Well, so we tried to explain what we thought had happened and our concerns about what was going on. We knew that his mind was under attack and had been altered, but we did not know why or how or what have you. So there was a lot of resistance and the social worker was most unsocial. . . . Nobody wanted to talk to us. . . . We really wanted to know what they were going to do, what kind of medicine they were going to give him. . . . And that was a real no-no. I mean . . . we . . . were the bad ones, the wild ones, because we were so questioning. . . . We wanted to know what was going on and nobody would tell us. And the other thing was, there was Jack in one of those little curtain things . . . and they wouldn't let us go be with him. . . . Jack was acting out. Well, big deal, he'd been acting out for the last three days. I mean, you know, he might calm down if we [could just] go in there. . . . They wouldn't let us in. . . . It was just mass confusion.

RETIRED SCHOOLTEACHER, *age sixty-two, father*

And a mother described an equally horrible experience the first time she had to hospitalize her daughter:

My child is hurting, really hurting [voice shaken]. And, I can't do anything to help her. I can't do anything to make it better for her. And she's not going to understand why these people are taking her and hurting her. Because, to her, everything is okay. She didn't do anything wrong. What has she done wrong to deserve people doing this to her? . . . It's totally out of her control what has happened to her [long pause]. . . . It breaks my heart to see her having to be restrained by four big huge men. They'd come and put her in restraint and she's crying and screaming, "Where is my mother?" "Why isn't my mother helping me?" It feels like my poor daughter saying, "Mom, if you love me, how can you let this happen to me?"

And yet, I'm doing it out of love, [I'm doing] things that are going to make her better. Getting her help, you know, 'cause that's the only way she's going to get better. I can't take her home and she doesn't understand this.... She talked about killing off the bad souls, so the good souls could return. And we had to have her hospitalized then, because I was afraid that she was gonna kill herself [*crying*] or kill people that she thought were bad souls.

RETIRED SECRETARY, *age fifty-eight, mother*

To the extent that these caregivers-to-be are blindsided by the first, sudden, and dramatically intense events signaling the onset of an episode of mental illness, they don't know what to think or feel. However, I should note that this reaction primarily characterizes the initial responses of spouses and parents. The situation is fundamentally different when one's entire childhood was dominated by the mental illness of a parent. After telling stories of family life that sounded exceedingly dysfunctional, individuals then typically declared that, as children, they knew no other world. They had somehow normalized their parenting of younger brothers and sisters while simultaneously coping with the needs of a mother or father who could not meet even minimal family obligations. For them, confusion about what to feel about themselves and ill family members often did not occur until they had acquired the perspective provided by adulthood and distance from their families of origin. Years of their adult lives were then spent reconciling mixed feelings about ill parents and deciding what their current obligations to care ought to be. Such emotional labor was also frequently done while mourning the loss of their childhood long after the fact.

From among the melange of inchoate, confused, and hurtful emotions that are part of coming to grips with a loved one's mental illness, one stands out as uniquely painful. It is the feeling of betrayal at having to hospitalize children against their will. One of the complexities surrounding the involuntary commitment of mentally ill persons is that they cannot be hospitalized unless it can be demonstrated that they are a risk to themselves or a danger to others.

Therefore, one of the most awful features of dealing with mentally ill individuals who cannot recognize the severity of their own difficulty is standing by helplessly while they decompose. Family members must simply wait for an episode to become so severe that they can then arrange for involuntary commitment.

Some of the most difficult-to-hear descriptions during interviews were given by parents, especially mothers, who had arranged for the police to remove a child from their home. Leslie, whose story begins this book, described through tears the scene of her barely clothed son being led away by police as he pleaded with them, "Please, just talk to my parents. They'll explain what an awful mistake you're making." Another mother, unwilling to collaborate in any process that would involve the police, hatched a plan to get her son into a hospital without having to issue a court order. Having been assured by a sympathetic family physician that a bed could be secured in a psychiatric ward, Eva then plotted with her boyfriend how to "lure" her son to the hospital. Despite her altogether humane intentions, the plan went badly awry:

So, anyway, I set it up and Jim [her boyfriend] helped me. . . . I said to him [Jim], "You've got to get Andy [son] out here [the hospital]." He called him up and he said, "Your mother called and she wants you to go see her. She's at a hospital up this way."

So he said that you . . .

That I was in the hospital and they were thinking about me staying and I wanted to see him first.

This was all a setup?

Yes. How else was I going to [get him into the hospital]? . . . I had this image, David, of some wonderful doctor to come in and sit with us for three days and tell this boy, "Look you have a lot of baggage," you know. So anyway, I got him to walk in the door. . . . He walked in the door and he looked at me and they closed those doors and he came in and said, "What's going on?" I said, "Andy, just come in and sit down," and he got very hostile, very angry. . . . I said, "Andy just sit down."

At this point did he know what was up?

He didn't know yet but he was getting hostile anyway. He was feeling it. So the guy [attendant] said, "Look, Andy, we just want to talk to you." [Andy says] "What is going on here? This is a trick." And he looks at Jim and he says, "Did you know about this?" . . . Anyway, David, for the next hour, he was just awful. [Andy] didn't want to answer any questions. He said, "I'm not talking to you. I'm getting out of here." And they are saying, "Andy, unless you talk to us you are not going to leave here." . . . He looked at me. He said, "Ma, don't do this to me. This isn't right." [She is sobbing.] I said, "Andy, you need help." I said, "I have to help you. We have to find out what is wrong." He said "Ma, don't do this to me." . . . They [doctors] came back in, and I said, "I've made a very big mistake. I want to leave and I want my son to leave." He [doctor] looked at me and he said, "He's staying." And I said, "No." My son stood up and he said, "We'll sue you." And he [doctor] said, "You're staying here and if your mother doesn't sign you in, we will."

So this all mushroomed into something much larger?

Oh my God, it was the biggest mistake I could have made. Everything went wrong from that point on, everything. First of all, Andy was out of his mind, out of his mind. He did not want me to sign the paper. I said, "Andy, don't you hear them, [unless I] sign the paper, they have the control." I was so afraid that he was maybe [so] sick that he would [never] come out. You know? And I wouldn't have the control. So I signed the paper. . . . I said, "Andy, please [cooperate]."

But he saw it as betrayal?

Oh yes. Oh David, I'll never forget his face going down the stairs. [He was saying], "I'll hate you for this." I left there a wreck. I hadn't slept the two weeks before planning this whole thing. My only consolation was that . . . "he's gotta get some help. He's gotta get some help."

REAL ESTATE BROKER, *age forty-five, mother*

Eva's story suggests another dimension of emotional anomie. During the early stages of what is eventually diagnosed as a mental illness, family members often doubt their own reading of the situation. They ask themselves: "Are my loved one's problematic behaviors only temporary? Will the situation resolve itself? Do I really need to involve health professionals in this matter? Is my spouse, child, sibling, or parent truly mentally ill?" If questions like these were not enough to produce and sustain great uncertainty, emotional anomie is sharply increased when the sick family member, and sometimes mental health professionals, cause caregivers to wonder whether *they* might, in fact, be the essential cause of the problem.

I figured I just wasn't a good person because I must be a failure [as a wife]. . . . I knew it was him, but I said [to myself], "No, maybe it isn't him. Maybe it's me."

DAY-CARE WORKER, *age fifty-five, wife*

↩

I felt like . . . life was totally out of [my] control. And especially [because] . . . there were so many times when he [son] would turn things around to make it look like I was the insane person [respondent laughs]. I mean, I'm just trying to help him, and then he would twist it and say, "I think you need a doctor."

SECRETARY, *age fifty-three, mother*

꒰

He [husband] convinced them [doctors] that I was the one who had
the problem, that I was the one who was overreacting and being
silly, and that it was me [respondent laughs]. . . . And so the woman
[doctor] then called me into the room and was saying, "Well, maybe
you're overreacting." And I was like, "Hold it." And so we left [the
emergency room]. I don't even remember what happened. Maybe
they set up an appointment for him to come back. I don't remember
what transpired.

CUSTOMER SERVICE REPRESENTATIVE, *age thirty-five, wife*

When madness first comes home, the only certainty is that *something* has gone horribly wrong. As the data thus far reveal, interviewees felt anxiety, fear, and, above all, sheer confusion. Such emotional anomie was further heightened by their impulse to deny that
the problem was mental illness. One mother recalled her reaction
to the initial phases of her daughter's illness by saying, "Denial is
a wonderful thing. [I tried to believe that] she's just a little off. She's
a little different." Another parent recalled her first reaction to the
mental illness label: "Mental illness. This could be years. This could
be friggin' years! Can you imagine how I felt? . . . I just said, "Oh
no, oh no, my son doesn't have a mental illness. My son isn't
psychotic."

Although the emergence of mental illness in a family devastates
everyone, the last several quotes suggest that women, mothers especially, are the most deeply affected emotionally. To be sure, the
data throughout this book lend support to the voluminous social
science literature on gender roles showing that the meanings men
and women assign to caregiving is affected by differences in their
socialization and by their social positions in society. You need only
take a walk to a local grade school at recess time to note differences
in the way that young children form friendship groups and play.
From a very early age boys and girls form sex-segregated friendship
groups that differ in size and content of activities. Little girls cluster

into relatively small, tightly knit groups in which a major activity is talk and the expression of feeling, whereas boys form into larger, more amorphous groups and largely engage in competitive games.[17]

From a very early age girls begin a learning process that centers their attention on human relations. Although there is a nascent "men's movement" in America with the goal of reducing gender inequalities and helping men to express their feelings and maximize their ability to experience intimacy, they still lag far behind women in their ability to talk about themselves and express emotion.[18] Men, in short, score high on sociability, but low on intimacy. While early socialization sets the stage for the nature of male and female relationships, that socialization is continually reinforced by women's actual locations in society. Especially relevant here, women nearly always function as the primary caretakers within families, doing the largely taken-for-granted, and thereby invisible, emotional work necessary for the daily well-being of family members.[19] We simply assume that it is women's "natural role" to provide emotional aid and social support for others, but especially their families. The normally invisible emotional kin work done by women becomes most readily apparent when families are in crisis.[20]

Somewhere along the line, troublesome family members were "officially" diagnosed as suffering from depression, manic-depression, or schizophrenia. Diagnosis is a pivotal moment in the lives of both patients and caregivers because both then typically embrace a medical version of what is wrong. As one parent put it, after diagnosis she now lived "in the nation of disability, the province of mental illness, and the village of manic-depression." The metaphor is apt since diagnosis thrusts both the caregiver and newly minted "patient" into a medical culture that defines the latter's troubles as disease. Moreover, since all cultures specify distinctive "feeling rules," commitment to a medical version of what ails a family member also provides caregivers with far greater clarity about appropriate emotions.[21] Because the prevailing medical view is that mental illnesses are brain diseases, healthy family members now feel obliged to treat their newly diagnosed parent, spouse, child, or sibling with the same love, understanding, sympathy, and compassion owed to any acutely ill family member.

Getting a Diagnosis

Although several respondents found it difficult to acknowledge that their family member was suffering from mental illness, most welcomed a firm diagnosis. After living for weeks, months, or even years in a kind of emotional limbo, it was comforting to have a name for their loved one's pain. If the problem could be clearly named, there was also hope that doctors could do something about it. However terrified they might be by the idea of mental illness and the specific diagnoses of depression, manic-depression, or schizophrenia, at least these categories objectified what was wrong and set in motion a course of medical treatment designed to relieve the problem.

After suffering from the emotional anomie already described, we can understand why respondents would say, "I loved getting the diagnosis. That was the best day of my life." Or, "I'll tell you [that] one of the best days of my life was when I got a phone call from the hospital telling me what was wrong with [my husband]." At this early point in a family member's illness, the caregiving role is normally embraced fully, enthusiastically, and optimistically. Family members care because they feel honest love and compassion for an ill child, spouse, parent, or sibling, but also because they know that it is their obligation to help. As reported in the last chapter, family members, at the beginning of things, gladly assumed their obligations to care.

> I can say that [it's] maybe 60% obligation. On the other hand, the fact that I do something because I'm obliged to do it, it does not mean that I do it only for that reason. I also love my mom. So, it's very mixed. It's something I know I have to do. But, that feeling

does not [come from] a superior being which tells me, "Ah! You
have to do that." It's nothing like that. Simply put, this is my situation and I have to handle it.

SALESMAN, *age thirty, son*

To genuinely care for another person presumes efforts to empathize with them, to feel what they feel, to try to see the world
from their standpoint, to "take their role."[22] Of course, all role-
taking is approximate since we can never fully understand what
another person is experiencing. From the outset, healthy family
members feel the unique contingencies of dealing with a mentally
ill person. The problem of accurate role-taking is dramatically magnified in the mental illness case if one has never experienced the
intense isolation, hopelessness, and despair of depression, the feelings of grandiosity during a period of hypomania, or the terror
accompanying paranoid delusions.[23] It is hard enough for a healthy
individual to empathize with a person who suffers from a physical
illness they themselves have never experienced. It is quite another
thing to understand a person whose mind is thoroughly inaccessible. However much they read about their family member's diagnosis
or tried to talk with them about their feelings, efforts to role-take
were incomplete and tremendously frustrating:

I don't understand it. I get absolutely frantic. I try to find out from
her [daughter] why she doesn't want to live.... She said to me,
"God won't give me cancer and I don't deserve to live so I have to
kill myself." And I'm thinking, "Why do you ... want God to give
you cancer?" And she said, "Because I don't deserve to be happy."
And I'm thinking, "Why?" And, of course, I get off the phone [and
then] I'm immediately back on the phone to the doctors to find out
how do I respond to this. What do I say to her?

HOMEMAKER, *age seventy-two, mother*

↜

One of the things she [wife] would say to me [is] "You don't understand what I'm going through. You belittle what I have here." In

this time period I came to the realization that "You're right, I don't understand and I never will. . . . I could never understand what you're going through, but I can definitely try to empathize and try to take my worst day when I feel bad and try to magnify ten or one hundred times and even that doesn't do any good."

SALESMAN, *age forty-two, husband*

The importance of role-taking in efforts to understand an ill family member once again prompts a comment about gender roles. An interesting body of literature indicates that the capacity to accurately see the world from the perspective of others, to empathize with them, varies systematically by social position. In particular, role-taking ability varies inversely with the degree of power associated with a person's social position.[24] Put plainly, some persons "make" roles and others are more constrained to "take" roles. Within the context of the family, Darwin Thomas and his colleagues demonstrate that fathers are less accurate role-takers than mothers.[25] Other studies show that women are more able than men to assess the subtle nonverbal cues reflecting another person's feelings.[26] Such research casts doubt on the pervasive and commonsense notion that women are, by nature, more tuned into the feelings of others. Rather, the greater role-taking ability of women may be rooted in the fact that they generally occupy less powerful positions than men, positions that demand a greater attentiveness to the wishes, feelings, and concerns of those more powerful than themselves.[27]

Were I to do an actual word count to determine the frequency with which respondents spontaneously described particular emotions, frustration would likely top the list. Caregiver frustration remained high at all points in the course of a family member's illness. As you will see, frustration sometimes became coupled with anger and resentment. Shortly after diagnosis, however, the frustration was linked primarily to a caregiver's inability to role-take with a person they wanted very much to understand and to help. Even though they could not fathom what it was like to be mentally ill, they remained optimistic and hopeful that they could get beyond a family member's initial episodes of illness. They believed, or tried to believe, that a combination of psychotropic drugs, talk therapy, and their own demonstrations of love, sympathy, and compassion would shortly resolve a solvable problem.

> We didn't have any understanding [of] how the illness works in terms of regaining one's focus and how much stress one can take. . . . And sometimes it takes so much time [to see improvement]. [You have to] take a day at a time. So, I mean we had . . . rather high expectations about how fast things were going to go and how much he was going to be able to do.
>
> RETIRED SCHOOLTEACHER, *age sixty-two, father*

↜

> The depth and breadth of love know no boundaries and I will cling to hope at all costs. To interfere with hope is the ultimate sin.
>
> PHYSICAL THERAPIST, *age forty-nine, mother*

The last person's heartfelt claim that "the depth and breadth of love know no boundaries" deserves expansion. Nearly everyone spoke of love for a suffering family member. It was, however, parents who most frequently and eloquently articulated the depth of their love. Such expressions often accompanied graphic descriptions of children when the illness had rendered them most helpless, vulnerable, and powerless. As an example, Anne, who has two children suffering from manic-depression, spoke of the hospital scene shortly after her son tried to commit suicide.

After swallowing a package of Benedryl, a common antihistamine bought over-the-counter, Jay was found in a groggy state and brought to a local hospital. When Anne arrived, she found him in a unit "one step down from intensive care." "He was sitting there wired to the EKG machine because his heart did have some arrhythmia." When Jay saw his mother, "he burst into tears . . . and so it was easy to interpret that he didn't want to die. . . . He just didn't like the way he was living." Later in the interview I asked

Anne, "Do you feel that all this extraordinary turmoil has deepened your relationship with your kids?" This question provoked the most emotion during our talk. Anne became teary and choked with feelings as she tried to answer. This is what she said:

> It opens up a dimension of love. We rarely touched. Jay still doesn't like being touched. And I thought I loved him [but] when I saw him at the [names hospital], with those EKG leads, the tears just burst forth and it was a different love. It was just overwhelming. You feel the affection, but it goes into a depth that you may never have known you are capable of. That's what I found. I thought I knew I loved my kids, but at that moment when they were so sadly afflicted, the depth was just . . . there was a purity. The sadness was a dimension, but there was [also] a feeling of love. You have the love that you felt [before] but it just expands to fill a space that you never even knew existed. . . . It's [a love] closer to truth. . . . I wouldn't want to have this [the tragedy of depression] visited on people, but I believe that I've had some special moments that other people don't have. . . . There's probably a better word than beauty. . . . I knew that truth was a factor in it [but there is also] a certain honesty. It was a very unguarded emotion. . . . I grew up in a household with a lot of mixed messages and never was able to trust my own emotions. But this one came without any [difficulty]. . . . To truly feel my own capacity to love, which I had not felt before, is liberating.
>
> NURSE, *age fifty, mother*

The emphasis of this section has been on the positive emotions of love, empathy, compassion, and hope because these are the ones most powerfully felt shortly after someone is formally diagnosed with depression, manic-depression, or schizophrenia. I suspect that caregivers will feel these same emotions during the early stages of *any* serious illness. These are the emotions one is "supposed" to feel when someone is first stricken with serious illness. In the case of mental illness, though, other more negative feelings also begin to creep into a caregiver's consciousness early on. These more ominously negative emotions, like worrisome storm clouds on a distant horizon, are linked to the realization that a mentally ill person cannot fulfill the usual requirements of the "sick role."[28] The "emotional economy" of sympathy is rooted in a norm of distributive justice that demands reciprocity in sympathy exchanges.[29] We normally expect patients to respond to care with expressions of gratitude and cooperative behavior. However, instead of making earnest efforts to get well and feel grateful for the care and concern they receive, emotionally ill people often treat family caregivers with disdain.

> He was reaming me out the other day. I mean, [he was] beating on me so terribly. I went there [his apartment] Saturday and this kid just wouldn't let me in. I bought him a bunch of things. He didn't want them. He threw them out in the street.
>
> REAL ESTATE BROKER, *age forty-five, mother*

↜

> I can't even imitate the tone of voice that she talks to me in. It's the tone of voice more than just the words that slices through you.
>
> GRADE SCHOOL TEACHER, *age forty-eight, mother*

↜

> He would just lash back at me. You know, it's none of your business if I take my medication. It's none of your business how often I am taking it or if I am taking it too much. . . . I would always be wondering if he was taking it because of the way that he was behaving, if maybe he was taking it all at once instead of . . . spacing it out throughout the day. . . . I would question him about that and [was told] it was none of my business. I would ask him at night when he was home, "Did you take your medication?" Again, "It's none of your business."
>
> SECRETARY, *age fifty-three, mother*

↜

Very depressed people are often very irritable and they say cruel things. My mother is worse with that. I think it's that mentally ill people . . . often act inappropriate or cruel or . . . aren't really there, aren't really tuned into what is going on. And they don't express . . . gratitude.

INSURANCE ADMINISTRATOR, *age forty-six, mother*

Rebuffs of the kind just described can be tolerated as long as they are seen as temporary manifestations of mental illness. Feelings of love, empathy, compassion, and sympathy shape the emotional terrain as long as caregivers believe that proper family and medical treatment will shortly fix the problem. When a husband, wife, son, daughter, mother, or father fails to respond to the family's and medicine's care, respondents begin to harbor more negative feelings. The eventual recognition that a family member's illness may well continue long into the future provokes feelings of intensified sorrow, but also of anger and resentment. In turn, the emergence of these unwelcome feelings calls forth the need for more deliberate emotion management. In the extreme case, caregivers had to reconcile hating someone they also love.

Perceiving the Permanence of Illness

Each Wednesday evening at 7 P.M., about twenty-five people arrive at the Family and Friends support group. It is interesting to observe that within the last six months a number of the spouses of ill wives or husbands, believing that their concerns are sufficiently distinctive, have created a group separate from the one now attended largely by parents and a few children and siblings. In both groups, though, there is a core of "regulars" who have been attending faithfully. Every week there are also a number of people wearing blue rather than red name tags, indicating that they are "first-timers." They are frequently referred to the group shortly after their first encounter with mental illness and, thus, are often suffering greatly from emotional anomie. During the two hours of "sharing and caring," one of the typical group dynamics is for caregiving "veterans" to socialize the "rookies."

Often, after newcomers give an account of their relatively brief history with an ill family member, they ask questions that are clearly prompted by the wish to know whether their experiences, behaviors, or feelings are idiosyncratic. Like social scientists new to the field, they wonder about the generalizability of their initial observations and perceptions. How usual is the number of medications taken by their loved one, the number of hospitalizations they have had, the frequency of their automobile accidents, their inability to hold jobs, their dismissal of doctors, the hostility they have been expressing at home, or their complete denial of the illness? They also want to know if they will ever have some relief from their unremitting anxiety, fear, bewilderment, sadness, frustration, and confusion. After a particular story is told or question asked, a veteran will often call for a show of hands: "How many of you have been through that?" All the old-timers raise their hands, nod knowingly at each other, and then, one by one, help to comfort newcomers by sharing a fundamentally similar story.

For troubled people to learn that they are not alone in their feelings and experiences is, indeed, one of the great values of support groups of all sorts. However, newcomers also learn something from veterans that visibly upsets them. They literally wince, shake their heads in disbelief, and sometimes audibly gasp when they learn that many of the regulars have been dealing with the ill person in their life for years, sometimes decades. Although the talk of the regulars is peppered with optimistic references to new drugs, new treatments, and the progress made by a loved one, their expressions of hope seem fundamentally contradicted by their own biographies. The folks wearing the blue tags have to entertain the possibility, often for the first time, that there will be no quick solution to the problem. Whether or not they have been the beneficiaries of a support group's collective wisdom, nearly all our respondents eventually had to incorporate into their thinking the likely permanence of their child's, parent's, sibling's, or spouse's illness.

When I was married . . . after all those years of realizing nothing was
going to change, [that] I was going to be married to somebody who
was mentally seven or eight years old and I was going to have to
care for three children instead of two, it was like, "I can't deal with
this anymore," and we divorced. Now I have a son who *I can't
divorce* [said with emphasis]. It's very frustrating that this may be
the way it's going to be. Here I am with that life [again], you know.

HOME HEALTH AIDE, *age forty-four, mother*

↜

I think, maybe over the first year, the first eight–nine months, my
feeling was that once she [daughter] came out of the coma and once
she went to [names hospital] that she was going to come out and
that she was going to be all right. That this was going to go away.
. . . And I think as we worked through . . . that first year, that was
my feeling. Then . . . when Dr. Johnson said that she needed long-
term hospitalization, and she went in . . . then I realized, okay, this
is it.

HOMEMAKER, *age seventy-two, mother*

The realization that a family member's mental illness may never
go away is a crucial identity turning point in the caregiving career
because it forces to the surface of consciousness an array of emotions that previously may have been only dimly felt. Now, caregivers
must surrender to the difficult reality that the expectations, aspirations, and hopes they had for the ill person in their life are unlikely to be realized. Parents, in particular, find it hugely painful to
let go of their dreams for their children. Because mental illness may
not erupt until late adolescence or early adulthood, parents have
spent years anticipating each of the usual life markers that ordinarily await bright, happy, intelligent, and creative children—high
school graduation, college, marriage, interesting work, having children. For many, coming to grips with their children's gross unhappiness and the knowledge that their life opportunities will be greatly
foreshortened by mental illness produces a profound sadness, a feeling of pervasive grief at having lost a child.

So bit by bit we lowered the expectations. . . . As things go on it's like somebody takes pieces of her and throws them away. Pieces of her keep disappearing over the years. More pieces of her disappear. She starts out whole and perfect and beautiful and over time pieces fall off. . . . And the older she got . . . I mean, I cannot bear to walk into [names high school]. I cannot bear it. It's too painful. [Other] people are graduating high school and going to proms. A couple of months ago my mother . . . came to visit and we went to Filene's. My mother wanted to buy her a birthday present and we ended up [looking at] prom gowns and I had to leave the store and sit in my car and weep. And I wasn't just weeping about the prom. It was the prom that opened the door for everything.

PHYSICAL THERAPIST, *age forty-nine, mother*

⤳

They would literally put her in a padded room next to the nurse's desk and when I would show up to see her . . . it was almost as if she curled up into my lap again—she didn't literally, but it was almost as if [she did]—and wanted to be touched and held. . . . Before she ran away, her hair had been very long but she had shaved it except for a patch on top. The nurses were a little wary when I asked for scissors. . . . I can still feel those moments as she curled up against the wall and I knelt next to her and I trimmed [her hair]. For those ten minutes she was my little girl and then she was somebody I didn't know again.

GRADE SCHOOL TEACHER, *age forty-eight, mother*

But the sense of profound loss is certainly not felt only by parents, as these comments illustrate:

If you are involved with anyone who has suffered from depression and you have a close enough relationship to them, I don't see how you cannot be very emotional about the situation. . . .Seeing it firsthand, it was just really hard on me. . . . I just felt like I lost a mom. You know? There is a chunk out of my life that was just no longer there. It was like this big void and I had to somehow fill it myself. You know, and I had to . . . grow up all of a sudden and I didn't necessarily feel . . . ready for it. . . . I felt so alone and by myself. . . . I felt like it was almost like role reversal; an eighteen-year-old kid taking care of someone that . . . is supposed to be taking care of you.

RESEARCH ASSISTANT, *age twenty-three, daughter*

⌐

It's an immense grief. It's an immense loss. I have friends that have relationships with their dads, where they call them up and ask them for advice, [relationships] where they're capable of confiding things in their dads. I've never had that experience—someone who could provide a role model for relationships. Do you know how many emotionally unavailable men I dated? It had a major impact on my relationship life as an adult. The only people I knew how to interact with . . . was someone who was really not available to me. It's really sad.

PHOTOGRAPHER, *age thirty-five, daughter*

A family member's enduring mental illness requires that caregivers not only radically revise downward their expectations for the ill person, but also that they ratchet down their own life expectations. For example, a young woman whose interview exuded compassion for her husband still felt anger that her own doctoral studies were being derailed by his inability to work and his need for constant care. One of his hospitalizations forced her to drop a class and she admitted to being "pissed off" and "feeling a weird anger," even though "it's not his fault per se." A husband, while acknowledging that his wife's hospitalization "was no picnic," began to resent that "the focus was always on her and her illness and it wasn't on me and what I've been doing to keep the family afloat and things like that." Caregiving to persons who are not getting better, who are unable to express gratitude for the help given them, and whose illness constrains one's own life creates great frustration. Frustration, in turn, breeds anger.

Their increasing isolation is surely one source of a caregiver's frustration. As their role extends for months or years beyond a family member's first episode, caregivers inhabit an increasingly constricted world dominated by the chronicity of mental illnesses, the often unreasonable demands placed on them, and the feeling that few people understand their own turmoil. Sometimes they respond by fundamentally reconstructing their social circles. One woman commented that she "[didn't] identify with normal people anymore," that she "cannot go to a cocktail party and talk nonsense, trivial conversation [but] will be with my Alliance [Alliance for the Mentally Ill] friends in a second." A mother who no longer attends such groups as the local PTA explained, "I've separated myself from them and I live in the nation of the wounded. I deal with my lowered expectations by looking for people who also gave up their expectations." The problem, however, is that caregivers can never fully separate themselves from the expectations and moral judgments of those who know little about the contingencies of caregiving.[30]

> Some people I don't know very well, like a neighbor down the street
> . . . my mother shows up on her doorstep and says, "I have no food."
> [The neighbor] will call and leave a message and say, "Go get your
> mother some food." Or my mother . . . doesn't have any friends or
> anyone to talk to but this one woman who, every once in a while,
> I'll hear from. . . . I don't really know how my mother even knows
> her, but she leaves a message: "I'm just calling to tell you, your
> mother's really sick so could you get her some help, thank-you," and
> [then she] hangs up. . . . People who have no understanding of men-
> tal illness really just think that the reason she is so sick is because
> you are not taking care of her.
>
>   ACCOUNTANT, *age thirty-five, daughter*
>
>   ↰

At that point I had nowhere to go and I had no support and I had no one listening to me. I had no family. My own mother was like,

"Stay with him" [husband]. My mother watched him smack me and I smacked him back for the first time, thinking my mom is going to think that I am this powerful woman, that I don't take that shit. It was the first time that I ever smacked him back and my mother said, "Next time you do something like that, I am going to have to call the police on you. That is just not a way for a woman to behave." And I was just like cross-eyed, like [what are you talking about]? And I . . . remember I spent a lot of time with just [that] kind of look on my face with a lot of people, you know? People would see that phase [of my life] and think "Sandy's being a bitch." They didn't see what made me turn into . . . being cold and demanding. It was my need to control this crazy environment.

STUDENT, *age twenty-five, wife*

As weeks become months or years, caregivers nearly always come to feel greatly frustrated by the persistent, ongoing trauma of mental illness. They find it harder to muster the compassion felt during the early stages of the illness. It is also harder for them to avoid feelings of anger and resentment. Partly because respondents typically tell their stories in a linear, chronological fashion, the feelings of anger and resentment do not surface until late in the interviews. It may also be uncomfortable to admit such negative feelings to a interviewer who might be yet another person ready to judge them harshly. Eventually, though, no caregiver story is complete until these feelings are expressed. Anger was often first voiced when respondents complained that their ill family member would not comply with medical treatment.

I got very angry at my father, not so much the first year when he had the breakdown. . . . When I got really angry was last year when I was moving into this [new law] office. We had been through [it] all [with him] last summer and I wanted to sit there and go, "Hey, listen, you are being really selfish now, okay? You are having these little episodes. You are not doing what everybody is telling you to do. You are not following what people are recommending." . . . He'd take the medicine, but he wouldn't do anything else. I said, "The medicines are [only] part of it." And he'd sit there with the "Woe is me, woe is me, I am taking these medications," and I said, "Listen ... nobody is saying it isn't awful. I am sure these medicines are making you feel terrible." [But] I was furious. I was so angry. I just wanted to say, "Will you just stop?" ... The pity was gone.

LAWYER, *age thirty-three, daughter*

〜

I have seen him [husband] at times go weeks without bathing or [doing] all of the things that could lead up to being out on the street by yourself. So, I do know it's for the long haul and I am willing to stick it out. ... We, together, really try. I mean, really [try] hard. I guess that is one of the things, you know, back to the question of why would you stick it out or what are the boundaries. ... Maybe it is, if he ever really stopped trying [I would leave]. Even when he was suicidal he didn't stop trying.

GRADUATE STUDENT, *age twenty-eight, wife*

When interviewees admitted to powerfully negative feelings, they nearly always offered the disclaimer that what disturbed them was not the person, but the person's illness. Because most of those interviewed believed that mental illness was a biochemical brain disease, it made sense to draw the illness/person distinction. However, such a dichotomy is also an invaluable tool for doing the emotion work required when a person has distressingly negative feelings toward a loved one. The person/illness distinction was mentioned in virtually every interview, but was unfailingly invoked whenever the word "hate" entered the conversation. The following comments are particularly instructive since they illustrate both how the person/illness distinction is used and the palpable residue of ambiguity about what a caregiver might legitimately hate.

It's one of those things that sounds sort of probably corny, but it's the thing that you hate her [mother's] illness, but you don't hate her. And I hate what she has done to us and the hell that she has

put us through. . . . I don't think that I hate her. You know, I probably . . . there's probably some degree of hating her. It feels like that,
but I think that it's more hating the illness. . . . I try to tell myself
that it's not her too. . . . You know, you're looking at her and saying,
"Well yuh, I hate you," but it's not I hate *you*. It's I hate what you
have done. I hate what you are doing. You know, I hate the illness.
. . . Your first reaction is to do that [hate them], but then . . . I guess
. . . you have to realize that it's really not them.

ACCOUNTANT, *age thirty-five, daughter*

↜

Sometimes I hate her, but mostly I don't hate her. Mostly I'm angry
at what she does. I mean, I'm angry at the behavior. I don't hate
her. I hate the behavior and I'm angry at the behavior. You know, I
hate that she took off and left me and I'm furious at her that she
took off on her eighteenth birthday and didn't call me for a week
and I thought that she was dead in a ditch. I am so angry at her
that she could do that to me. And the therapist keeps saying, "She
didn't do it to you, she just did it. . . . You weren't a piece of this
picture at all. She just did this." But it's going to take me a really
long time to forgive her for that. . . . I'm angry at her for doing that
but I don't hate her because it's the illness, it's not her. But there
have been moments when I hated her. Every time she does something bad I call it the illness now, you know. . . . They tell me she's
really sick and they tell me she's really severe. So it's easier to call
this illness than to call this asshole adolescent behavior, you know?

PHYSICAL THERAPIST, *age forty-nine, mother*

↜

I don't think that I have ever gone to hate. There is plenty of resentment, more for the situation that it puts us in than at her. Probably more at the disease than at her, but [then] she is the disease.

SALESMAN, *age forty-two, husband*

You have already seen how difficult it is for caregivers to draw
boundaries throughout the entire course of another person's

mental illness. However, boundary-drawing becomes a still more delicate task once the permanence of illness becomes apparent. By then, family members have already felt the pain of losing their once well child, spouse, parent, or sibling. By the time they have traversed the emotional journey from anomie to compassion to periodic feelings of hatred, they also realize that they are in danger of losing themselves. Distancing themselves from a person they love, even as a measure to save themselves, is emotionally wrenching.

Acceptance

One of the tricky things about formulating an analysis that focuses on change and process is that each respondent is to some degree "in a different place" in their caregiving history. Just as in the MDDA support group, the people interviewed for this study range from those who are caring for someone only recently diagnosed to those whose lives have been circumscribed by mental illness for a decade or more. Thus, while everyone faces the same problem of balancing a sense of obligation with the proper level of caregiving involvement, time spent at the task leads to a different calculus of care. Within the Family and Friends group, for example, it is the veterans who most enthusiastically endorse the Four Cs mantra— "I didn't cause it. I can't control it. I can't cure it. All I can do is cope with it." Such a proscription has a Buddhist-like motif because those who can truly act on it in their daily life have learned that suffering substantially diminishes with its acceptance. Efforts to fix another person's illness are typically abandoned when caregivers finally understand that, however much they care, they cannot control their family member's illness and that by caring too much they are losing themselves. First, this is how they spoke of lack of control:

> I've got to read you something. I've got to read you this. [She reads from a paper she has written]: "There is a special place in my coun-

try called the garden of acceptance. It's very difficult to find and no one is able to give directions on how to get there. In fact, each villager reaches the garden by a different route. The only common feature in the journey is the letting go of control. As long as one seeks to hold on to control of their illness or disease they cannot enter into the garden of acceptance. Only when you lay this particular burden down do you find the elusive peace which this garden provides." And right now I've cried a lot because I'm giving up the last piece of control.

PHYSICAL THERAPIST, *age forty-nine, mother*

It took me two years to understand what it meant to have a daughter who was mentally ill. I worked that through for two years. I accepted the fact that I had no control over her; that I couldn't keep her safe. This is the acceptance. The acceptance has not been so much that she is mentally ill. The hardest acceptance is that I couldn't keep her safe. I couldn't prevent her from being a jerk or from being out of control or from making bad decisions. I had no control over her. . . . It took me two years to get there. I worked hard to get there. It doesn't change the fact that she's been hard to deal with sometimes. It just means that . . . the struggle that I do is different. The struggle that I do with her right now feels smaller and less emotionally tangled.

GRADE SCHOOL TEACHER, *age forty-eight, mother*

Now, this is how they spoke about losing their identities:

If I could not maintain my own self-identity, if my identity was so caught up . . . into this aspect of him [husband] that it was crippling me, I could no longer do this. And the two times I've bailed out, or temporarily wanted to be separated, was exactly for these issues. I felt like he was sucking all of my spiritual [and] emotional energy right out of me. . . . I left him at Christmas time because I just couldn't take the negativity any more. It was the hardest, it was the most difficult, the best thing I ever did. [I told him], "I love you, but I can't live with you anymore. I have absolutely no problem that I love you, but I just can't be pulled down by this anymore. I have to take care of me."

NURSE, *age fifty, mother*

⤶

I guess I have seen with both my mother and my sister what a devastating effect it [depression] has on the people around them. So I just don't want that around me very much. I don't feel like I am strong enough to withstand it. I guess I feel some people would be, [but] I am not. And I don't want to be destroyed by it.... Even now I feel ... with my mother sometimes [that] her desire is to destroy me.... I know [this] isn't really true, but I feel if she could completely absorb me and take all of my energy and life in her illness, she would. This is sort of what she is after and I have to protect myself from that.

INSURANCE ADMINISTRATOR, *age forty-six, daughter*

⤶

I don't want to have all of these relatives who are sick and I don't want this to be my identification and my persona. I don't want this to be the sum of who I am—sick relatives.

TECHNOLOGY LICENSER, *age thirty-three, sister*

Although caregivers can cognitively understand that their efforts to control are fruitless and that their identities are being undermined, the decision to back away from the obligation to care remains, nevertheless, emotionally very difficult. This is partly so because respondents have deeply internalized conceptions of what it means to be a moral person. One daughter allowed that she "could walk away from it," but did not want to meet her God without having done "everything that I could have, everything that was reasonable for me to do." A woman, married for more than thirty years, while acknowledging that she no longer loved her husband, also said, "I feel badly for him. He's a human being. I've known him most of my life. You can't throw people away." A husband who felt he was able "to keep an arm's length" from his suicidal wife also described himself as "a person who keeps agreements." And a daughter who "realized years ago that [she] couldn't save [her] parents," still felt enormous guilt:

> I feel guilty for being angry. I am guilty for blaming them. I am guilty for feeling the way I feel. I feel guilty for the fact that, although I know rationally there is no basis for it, I may be happy. I feel guilty towards my father that I am venturing on a successful career [as a lawyer]. I feel guilty that I am more successful [now] than ... he was at [his] height.
>
> LAWYER, age thirty-three, daughter

As you might expect, I heard a great deal about trying to let go without guilt.

> I can be there and I can be supportive, but the bottom line is that there is plenty of opportunity for her to kill herself and if she wants to she can. I mean, I can't be with her twenty-four hours a day, seven days a week, for the rest of our lives.
>
> SALESMAN, age forty-two, husband

↩

> Last night, her [daughter] stepsister was over, and they were watching TV. . . . Her stepsister has a tendency to drink, so I've already told Joyce that if she chooses to drink, that's her choice. But, my choice is that I'll be washing my hands of the whole thing, because you can't drink and take the kind of medication [she's taking]. And if she chooses to do it, she chooses to get sick again. And I [also] said, "Joyce, you're an adult. I don't want to have to be coming out and cleaning your apartment, sorting through your bills, calling your creditors, and doing all that. I don't want to do it." . . . I mean, I absolutely refuse to pamper her. I said, "No, mommy is not going

be here to take care of you. I'll help when I can, but only if you're helping yourself. Because if you're not going to do anything to help yourself, I can't help you."

RETIRED SECRETARY, *age fifty-eight, mother*

Believing that they cannot control another person's illness and that ultimately they are not primarily responsible for the fate of a sick child, spouse, or parent leads some to a kind of resigned acceptance. A few interviewees, however, have achieved a more affirmative kind of acceptance. Earlier I described the chronic sorrow caregivers feel as they try to relinquish their hopes and aspirations for a child, parent, or spouse lost to mental illness. Once beyond their profound loss, some people come to a deep admiration and respect for their family members who bravely struggle with the unimaginable pain of mental illness. They no longer measure their loved one in terms of pre-illness potentials now gone. Their new aspiration is to help them to become as happy and productive as their sickness will allow.

You know, I just want him [to be] happy and stable. I mean, at this point I don't have any [grand] expectations. He is a wonderful kid. He's pure. I just look at him as this innocent, good kid. This is how I see him and it doesn't matter to me what he does in life. . . . I just want him to stabilize, accept his illness, and just get on with his life.

SECRETARY, *age fifty-three, mother*

↬

I'm just in awe of Jack and his abilities to deal with circumstances and to keep a kind of patience, a kind of perspective, and a willingness to work with things, things that are not his first choices, needless to say. . . . [There is still] intense sadness that Jack has to do this, has to have this. I mean, that will bring tears to my eyes, but [also] an incredible admiration for his attitude toward dealing with it.

RETIRED SCHOOLTEACHER, *age sixty-two, father*

↩

Coping with it . . . is to accept the person for who they are and love them for who they are and develop a positive relationship with them. I have heard some parents in the group (MDDA) who cannot get over the stigma of mental illness. And [then] you see the ones who are more developed in their thinking saying, "I'm just glad to have them around and I'll take them on whatever level I can have my kids."

TECHNOLOGY LICENSER, *age thirty-three, sister*

Of course, "to accept [a] person for who they are and love them for who they are" is the most unalloyed kind of acceptance and love because it is given unconditionally. The words of these individuals remind us of an earlier caveat not to shortchange the role of love, along with a profound sense of obligation and responsibility, in producing caregiving commitment to severely ill people. Finally, although it would be wrong to romanticize sickness, I feel persuaded that a family member's life-altering illness can sometimes provide caregivers the opportunity to feel a depth of acceptance for a child, spouse, parent, or sibling that might not otherwise be possible.

Efforts to deal with a mentally ill family member arouse especially strong emotions because people suffering from depression, manic-depression, or schizophrenia pose such distinctive threats to the order and coherence of daily life. The behaviors of mentally ill people are nearly always incomprehensible. They may also be socially objectionable, threatening, and dangerous. In addition, the mentally ill are often unable to understand their own circumstance, are sometimes unwilling to accept medical diagnoses, may not comply with medical treatment, and frequently cannot express appropriate gratitude for the care accorded them. These contingencies require that family caregivers engage in especially arduous interpretive efforts to make sense of their feelings.

Moreover, there is a pattern to the way caregivers experience emotions over time. That is, the link between a family member's emotional illness and a caregiver's emotions has a decidedly historical dimension.

I identified four critical junctures in the parallel social trajectories of mentally ill people and their family caregivers. Prior to medical diagnosis, family members feel utterly bewildered by an ill person's behaviors and do not know how to react, behaviorally or emotionally. I used the term emotional anomie to describe this initial period in the joint career of ill people and family caregivers. Following diagnosis, caregivers make valiant efforts to empathize with their ill spouse, child, parent, or sibling, often believing that a combination of medical treatment and their own loving care will solve the problem. Once it becomes clear that a family member's illness is chronic and probably unsolvable, the kinder emotions of sympathy and concern typically recede and darker feelings of frustration, anger, and resentment surface. These negative emotions are especially likely to arise if caregivers come to believe that their sick family member is not assuming appropriate responsibility for getting well. Finally, some caregivers conclude that a person's illness is well beyond their control. Such a recognition may liberate them by legitimating their withdrawal without guilt.

Oddly, students of emotion have neglected the processes through which feelings in the present articulate with the past. The need to see any emotional expression in terms of a whole history of incidences and affects meets the test of personal introspection. For example, a worker's outburst of anger will ordinarily be connected to a complex history of perceived slights or ill treatment by colleagues or superiors. As therapists have always argued, displays of strongly negative emotions between spouses rarely reflect only the circumstances of the moment. Rather, such feelings, like solidified geologic formations, arise from an accretion of hurts, injuries, and perceived injustices built up over years. Equally, warm feelings and moments of tenderness between a husband and wife are inseparable from the marital history they have jointly produced. Although there are surely dramatic, time-limited moments of high emotion, an exclusive focus on the immediacy of feelings distracts attention from the importance of seeing emotions as emergent properties of a broader stream of social experience.

Greater attention to the historical properties of emotion evolution is important on theoretical grounds alone. However, studies that show how emotions shift in predictable ways through the life course of any important process may also have significant practical value. Just as I have shown that caregiver careers proceed through a predictable series of feeling frames, I presume that a wide range of important phenomena can be described the same way. For example, such an approach might be used to illuminate the emotions characterizing the different phases of social movements, political campaigns, undergraduate college careers, family-run businesses, marriages, or, for that matter, writing books. If we could know in advance the likely sequence of emotions in these and similar social processes, we could better prepare people who will experience them by choice or chance. In the end, though, a research agenda of the sort proposed here is required by the mandates of the sociological imagination itself. Emotions, like all social things, arise through the "interplay of man and society, of biography and history, of self and world."[31] Theories of emotion that do not attend to these connections are simply incomplete.

Taken together, Chapters 2 and 3 describe the two most general features of caring for family members with any illness. Healthy family members must try to establish appropriate obligation boundaries with an ill person and manage the emotions that arise predictably over the course of an illness. For reasons specified in these chapters, mental illness creates special complexities in performing these caregiving tasks. Through their own words, I have tried to portray some of the confusion, uncertainty, and ambiguity that arise as caregivers try to draw boundary lines and manage the painful emotions created by mental illness. However, not everyone feels the same obligations and emotions when a family member becomes sick with depression, manic-depression, or schizophrenia. As suggested at several points, parents, spouses, siblings, and children differ in the way they approach the burdens of caregiving. I choose to continue my conceptual story by describing these differences in Chapter 4.

FOUR

Family Ties

It's kind of hard to put [my feelings] into words. I mean I love my parents dearly and I love my brother, and I think you're raised to know what's right and wrong. And I do feel like your family comes first. But by the same token, how much . . . is realistic for a sibling to give up? Are you supposed to give up your life? And [give up] your career? I mean, [do you give up] your hopes? . . . And it's like where do draw the line? Just where do you draw the line? Do you do what's right for your family and just do it unselfishly? It's a hard thing. It's easy to say, "Yeah, I'd do anything for my family" until you really have to . . . until you are faced with it.

OFFICE MANAGER, *age thirty-seven, sister*

To reveal the character of moral obligations, I often ask the students in my Introduction to Sociology class, "What do you owe your parents?" After the initial silence such a question normally produces, someone eventually offers the opinion, "I owe my parents *everything*." Student might elaborate by describing their good home life and upbringing, adding that their parents did, after all, bring them into the world. Students also typically talk about the opportunities they have been given for a good education, stressing the sacrifices made by their parents for them. After a few declarations of this sort, I then ask just what they mean by "owing them everything." Does it mean that such important life decisions as choice of work, whom to marry, where to live, and the timing of children will be premised on their parents' wishes? "Well, no," the students are then likely to say. After a series of such questions, "owing them everything" becomes more cloudy and there is consensus only that they love their parents, want their respect, and have a generalized expectation that they will "be there for them" if mom and dad ever need help.

Since teaching should get students to see the complexity in the things they normally take for granted, I then purposely muddy up the conversation a bit by reading a scene from the movie *Guess Who's Coming to Dinner?* You may recall that this 1967 Sidney Poitier film is about the love affair between a black doctor and a white woman from a well-to-do family. The entire movie takes place at the girl's home on the occasion of the first meeting of the couple's parents. Although the girl's parents, played by Katharine Hepburn and Spencer Tracy, are "liberals," it is clear that they are, at the least, uncomfortable with the impending marriage. Most uncomfortable, though, is the doctor's father, a mailman. In one scene, father and son are alone together. With a sense of indignant self-righteousness, the middle-aged father expresses his outrage at his son's love affair. In abbreviated form, here is the father's "speech" and his son's equally angry response:

> FATHER: Son, you've got to listen to me. Now, I'm not trying to tell you how to live your life, but you never made a mistake like this before. . . . Have you thought what people would say about you? Why in sixteen or seventeen states you'd be breaking the law. You'd be criminals. And say they changed the criminal law, that don't change the way people feel about this thing. You know, for a man who always never put a wrong foot anywhere, you're way out of line boy.
>
> SON: That's for me to decide, man. So, just shut up and let me. . . .
>
> FATHER: You don't say that to me. You haven't got the right to even say a thing like that to me, not after what I've been to you. And you know that and I know that. Yuh, I know what you are and what you've made yourself. . . . You know I worked my ass off to get

the money to buy you all the chances you've had. You know how far I carried that bag in thirty years? Seventy-five thousand miles and mowing lawns in the dark so you wouldn't have to be stokin' furnaces and could bear down on the books. I tell you, there were things your mother should have had that she insisted go instead for you. And I don't mean fancy things. I mean a decent coat, a lousy coat. And you're going to tell me now that means nothing to you. . . .

SON: You listen to me. You say you don't want to tell me how to live my life, so what do you think you've been doing? You tell me what rights I've got or haven't got and what I owe you for what you've done for me. Let me tell you something. I owe you nothing. If you carried that bag a million miles you did what you were supposed to do. Because you brought me into this world and from that day you owed me everything you could ever do for me, like I will owe my son.

The juxtaposition of the students' initial pledges of owing their parents everything with Poitier's words expands our dialogue. Some students now agree that since their parents "chose" to have them, they are owed far more than they owe. Nearly always the conversation also reveals the distinctive norms of different cultural groups. If I am fortunate enough to have foreign students in my class, especially from East Asia, they describe a far heavier debt of obligation to parents than their American peers. If the conversation continues by considering the obligations of siblings and spouses, the students begin to see that a sense of obligation is situationally constructed and significantly determined by social status. Agreement eventually arises that parents have different obligations to children than children have to parents, and that the ties between siblings are more tenuous than those between parent and child. And because the relationship of spouses is socially constructed rather than bounded by blood, they are freer to leave each other's lives if the "going gets too tough."

This chapter looks at the strength of family ties, but departs from the earlier mode of data presentation. Although I have already provided modestly detailed descriptions of particular individuals, most of my earlier analyses depend on the comments of many respondents. Allowing lots of respondents to speak is an effective way to demonstrate patterns in the way caregivers think about their task. However, it is also important to preserve and honor the integrity of the stories I heard. A significant tension in presenting and analyzing in-depth interview materials is to reveal consistencies in the experiences of people while recognizing the distinctiveness of each person's narrative. To be sure, each of the sixty stories collected for this volume has its own flavor and tone. No two respondents face precisely the same contingencies as they try to work out the family problems generated by mental illness. The art of interviewing requires that one gather systematic data on features of the caregiving experience while being respectful of the uniqueness of each person's account. As part of my own obligation to those interviewed, I will use this chapter to tell a more complete version of three stories about caring and commitment.

Naturally, it would be problematic to generalize from three cases.[1] Each case contains details that have no duplicate elsewhere. Indeed, although the motif of this chapter will be to tell of three experiences in a more complete way than other formats allow, the accounts to follow are still too brief to capture the full range of incidences, emotions, and perspectives connected with their caregiving. Even the fifty- to eighty-page transcript covering a several-hour conversation can only capture the broad contours of a person's biography. I suppose that if each of the individuals I interviewed wrote book-length memoirs, the materials would still provide only an approximation of how living with a mentally ill person has transformed their lives. Still, the cases I choose to highlight in this chapter can push along our thinking about the way a person's relationship to an emotionally ill family member shapes his or her thoughts, feelings, and actions. This is so because I have strategically chosen these cases in the context of what I have learned by listening to all the people constituting this study. I feel confident that the stories I have selected reflect broad regularities in the way that children, siblings, and spouses view their obligations to sick parents, brothers or sisters, and partners, respectively.

From time to time, people who know that I have been working on this book ask me what I have been learning. The members of the MDDA support group have been especially interested in hearing what insights a sociologist has to offer after listening to them for more than three years. Sometimes I tell them what I have learned about changes in obligations and emotions over time. I might, though, also tell them that I have noted essential differences in the ways parents, mothers in particular, view caregiving obligations. I began this book by telling Leslie's story—a mother's story. Stories like hers let me half joke that mothers are on an entirely different caregiving planet. In general, though, parents display an unparalleled level of commitment to an ill child, often to the point of threatening their own emotional and physical well-being. Since Leslie and so many other parents have already spoken in earlier chapters, I will use the remainder of this chapter to let a child, a sibling, and a spouse speak more fully.

I maintain that it is the peculiar plight of children that they can make sense of the way a parent's mental illness has shaped them only years later. In particular, children feel a pervasive sense of having been betrayed by their parents and spend adult years trying to build identities stunted in childhood. Siblings typically have much lower levels of involvement than their parents in the lives of a sick brother or sister. During childhood, they often do not fully understand that their sibling's objectionable behaviors arise from a mental illness. As adults, they wonder whether a greater level of responsibility might have significantly altered the course of a brother's or sister's life. And spouses, more than other family members, feel that under certain conditions they might properly end the relationship altogether. However partial they might be, each of the stories to follow amplifies these broad themes.

What Do You Owe Your Parents?

Since one-third the respondents for this study were people I met through the MDDA support group, I deliberately sought to broaden my sample by recruiting individuals from other sources—referrals from interviewees and my own friends, students in my classes, audience members at public talks I give, and newspaper advertisements. Interviews with these people persuade me that the themes I have been discussing here cut across different populations of caregivers. Jason, a thirty-year-old artist with an ill mother and brother, called me after reading an ad I placed in a local newspaper. Our eventual conversation was fundamentally similar to the accounts of other children who grew up in a "madhouse." However, Jason's story is singularly unique in one striking way. He has been fleeing from his mother who "has a sort of stalking mentality." He told me at the outset of our talk, "I have to take extreme measures just to have a measure of control in my life." After a childhood that required him to "bury [his] feelings in order to be accepted," Jason is now struggling "to be connected with friends, to be connected with myself."

After a few preliminary demographic questions, I typically ask a person to tell me about the first moment it entered his or her consciousness that something was wrong with a family member. Although Jason acknowledged that, like all of us, his memories of childhood are reconstructed from an adult point of view, he replied that his mother "had her first breakdown when I was seven or eight. . . . I have memories of her practically hanging out of our fourth story window . . . yelling at ambulances as they would drive by, because we lived right across from a hospital. 'They are coming to take me away.' You know this kind of extreme paranoia." Confirming his earlier self-description as a person who "frames things in a visual way," Jason continued by saying, "With that particular image of my mother hanging out the window, I have a flash of a memory of . . . the room being very dark and [the] lights of the passing cars sort of projecting these long shadows along the ceiling. . . . I was feeling by myself, feeling very alone as a kid, looking at this room and my mother . . . [who was] acting very frantically." Trying to recollect traumatic events after nearly twenty-five years, Jason continued his description this way:

> I mean, even as I am talking about it . . . I don't know whether I am creating sort of a montage of a moment. . . . I don't know whether I am embellishing to some degree my mother being frantic and her yelling, you know, "They are coming to take me away." I mean, I know she did things like that and that stands out in my mind as a kind of memory. . . . I [also] have a memory of her coming home from something, I think it was work . . . and my brother and my father were like doing a math project in the hall and my mother came home and she was clearly very depressed and distraught and there was a palpable sense that something was wrong. I think she went into the bedroom and sort of shut the door behind her and my dad might have followed and that seemed to me as sort of the beginning of her descent. . . . I [also] remember my mother and my father having very drawn-out, loud yelling fights. . . . She is yelling at him and he yells back as just a way to create some kind of barrier, you know? . . . It did get physical at some point. We had this big hall mirror. . . . My dad threw her into the mirror and it shattered. . . . I don't remember if I was at the other end of the hall or in my room. I know it happened. I know I heard it. I think I might have seen it, but I am not sure. So, you know, all of these things are like shards, like the glass, like the mirror itself.

As the story of his childhood began to spill out, Jason kept returning to the twin themes that characterize the accounts of nearly everyone who grew up with a mentally ill parent—anger and abandonment. Children growing up in utterly chaotic households have the predicament of making sense of their own volatile emotions. Jason astutely commented that children simply do not have "adult tools like wisdom and maturity . . . stuff that just being older gives you to process the experience in an easier way." Perhaps even more than for his mother, Jason harbored animosity toward his father, who did little to validate his son's pain. As an example, Jason told me, "I would lock myself in the bathroom and basically pound the paint off the door and my father would say things like, 'You have to learn to control your anger.'" Rather than validating emotions that were appropriate for a child who was "really scared," these comments, Jason felt, created a sense of shame and guilt so powerful that they continue to shape his adult life. He recalled, "I think I was really hurt. . . . I think I was grieving. I was raging. I was in a lot of pain. . . . I don't think an eight-year-old can very easily make connections between their emotions and their life circumstances. . . . That was a big part of the problem."

One of the most awkward dilemmas for children of parents who are themselves consumed by mental illness, either as the sick person or the engulfed spouse, is that normal social roles are often inverted. With the same kind of insight that characterized his observations throughout our interview, Jason explained that "it is terrifying to a child when the parent needs to be nurtured. I mean, when you are eight, nine, ten, eleven years old it is terrifying to a child to have your parent helpless. . . . This is not the right role." Such a role reversal, Jason noted, is especially confusing in the case of emotional illness. "If parents go through a physical disability," he observed, "I'm sure the children are also angry. The parent cannot take care of you in the way that they could before. . . . [You say to yourself] 'Well, how could they?' When it is emotional and mental, it is harder to accept and to understand . . . to justify it." Jason then plaintively remembered, "I don't think as a kid I bought the idea that my mother was crazy . . . I wanted her to be my mother, you know. And I am sure that I tried a thousand different angles and approaches to get her to be my mother again and none of them worked."

Feelings of abandonment were greatly exacerbated when Jason's father left home. Having been told by a lawyer that he could gain custody of his two sons only by proving his wife's incompetence, Jason's dad saw no alternative except to leave the household. His father "would come in at night and sort of make sure that we were okay. . . . So, basically he wasn't sleeping there and he wasn't a part of the household. So, we weren't completely abandoned . . . in the sense that he was a presence. . . . But in terms of feeling terrified, my brother and I . . . had to go through this concentrated period of hell. . . . I think it was for months." Eventually, their father filed for divorce and got automatic custody when "my mother didn't appear for the court date."

After the two boys moved to their father's apartment, Jason's mother was periodically hospitalized where she was "given Thorazine and drugged out." Although his mother "has not to this day accepted that she has any kind of problems," she abandoned their old apartment "in her mania and in her terror," eventually ending up on the street. Some months after the two brothers left to be with their father, the three returned to their former, now unoccupied apartment to learn that it had been ransacked. With a sense of artistic irony, Jason described the emotional effect of the scene: "It was like the exclamation point after this very long, loud, traumatizing sentence!"

Her life on the streets was a turning point for both mother and children. For several years, Jason recalled, "We would get calls from my mother on the streets. . . . Sometimes she would just kind of cry or she would say, 'You know, I'm not crazy.' You know, 'Someone has poisoned me,' or 'This is all your father's fault.' " At first, Jason agreed to meet his mother in one or another public place, but, over time, felt that it was less hurtful to avoid his mother than to see her. Here's what might happen when they did meet:

My mother is and was the source of extreme trauma and pain, so my first reaction was, "I don't want to deal with that." But . . . on regular intervals, maybe once or twice a week for a period of time, and maybe going down to once or twice a month, and then maybe going down to a few times a year . . . my brother and I would go see her. We might meet at a coffee shop or something and it was mainly out of guilt and, yes, love. . . . But there is nothing that we could do

for her. That was the real frustration. And she would—even a nine
or ten or eleven year old kid—she would ask for money and we
would like meet at a cafe and she'd cry and she'd chain smoke and
drink her coffee and at some point it would escalate to a yelling or
a crying thing. It would be a scene and as a kid I would be scared
and embarrassed and I would basically want to get away. [Your] first
reaction is protection. I want to protect myself.... I mean, I obviously had to sort of disassociate. I had to separate myself from my
mother and separate my feelings for her because [otherwise] it would
be too painful.

Although realizing that "part of me was dead," Jason tried to
live the ordinary life of a teenager, a task partly accomplished by
keeping his sorrow private, by "repressing on all four cylinders,"
and by "getting some relief from sports." At a point, though, re-
pression and exercise simply could not contain the "the tremendous
anger and sadness [he] was carrying around." One evening, while
returning with friends via subway from a concert, Jason described
how he was overtaken by his emotions. "I just broke out in tears.
I couldn't control myself. I couldn't stop it. And I remember, there
was a guy sitting across from me on the train, an African-American
man [who] looked sort of destitute. He just said to me, 'You got
to let it all out. You got to let it all out.' I kind of heard it and I
was just wailing and feeling very ashamed." When he composed
himself, Jason realized that "the genie was out of the bottle" and
that his buddies had "found me out." The opposite reactions of the
two friends who witnessed Jason's "breakdown" confirmed both the
cost of expressing vulnerability so publicly and its potential for
solidifying human connections. Although he lost one of those
friends, the second, who came from "a divorced family," responded
with compassion and the disclosure of his own previously invisible
pain.

Questions of disclosure remain thorny for Jason, as they often
are for other family members of the mentally ill. Just how much
ought one to say about the intricacies of a life complicated by a

mother's mental illness? On the one hand, it is difficult to build meaningful relationships while withholding information about one's identity that is so central to one's sense of self. The disclosure of such information, however, may very well abruptly end potentially meaningful relationships. It would be shocking to tell a new acquaintance, "I have a family member who is mentally ill and [has] a stalking mentality. She is not dangerous, but will harass me and make my life difficult." I asked how he managed such information in the construction of the relationship with his current girlfriend of more than two years. Jason told me that "she is extremely patient and is a social worker, which helps." When they first met and began to exchange biographical information, Jason told her right away, "I have baggage.... I know everyone has baggage, but I have some pretty extreme things that have happened in my life." As a general strategy, he said, "I pace it out based on what is comfortable for me and what is comfortable for them."

As years passed, Jason increasingly distanced himself from his mother who "had fixated on [him] as the person that will rescue her." When she has been able to locate him, Jason's mother would call forty or fifty times a day "during her peak mania." Unable to live his life under those conditions, Jason has, in effect, gone underground. In response, his mother has gone to great lengths to find him, once hiring a search agency that used voting registration records to locate him in the Midwest. On a second occasion, she broke into the house of an aunt who knew his whereabouts. The break-in was successful. She found materials with his address, prompting Jason yet again to change jobs and states. Now, all bills are in his girlfriend's name, he avoids identification cards of all sorts, and told me, "I might ... get to the point where I have to change my name." Recently, he took a new job and had to contend with his supervisor's understandable incomprehension when told "I can't be on the net." He was obliged to write a formal letter explaining why having an e-mail address compromises his security. The letter worked, but only after he finally told a version of the story I am narrating.

Throughout most of our conversation, Jason mentioned his older brother Adam largely in passing. The two boys mutually lost their childhood in the devastating morass of their mother's illness. Aside from that absolutely life-shaping commonality, Jason saw himself as more artistic than Adam who always wanted to figure things out logically. Jason also thought that "my mother sort of clutched me and my dad sort of clutched my brother. My dad sort of protected my brother because my mother was [especially] cruel to him. . . . So, when my mother was out of the scene I kind of felt like my brother and my father were . . . this team and I was the odd man out." However, Jason also told me that "as the years went on [Adam] was pretty protective and understanding of me and very supportive and very proud in an open way." The biggest difference between the two boys, though, is that mental illness has now claimed Jason's thirty-three-year-old brother. Although Adam has been able to piece together work from time to time, his "delusions and rage" have repeatedly gotten him into trouble with the police and precipitated several hospitalizations. These days the brothers are most likely to speak after one of Adam's episodes.

I hadn't heard from him [in a while] and then I heard that he was arrested because he was sleeping in the post office and the police came by and kicked him out and he got into a fight with the policeman. . . . Then I knew that something seriously was wrong and I just heard all of these stories. . . . I wouldn't hear from him. . . . He would call my dad or I would hear from a relative or a friend that he was in a mental hospital or he was in jail for . . . one kind of authority issue or another. And that kind of happened with more and more consistency and regularity and he hasn't held down a job. . . . He has basically been either in a jail system or in the mental health system . . . for the past four or five years. . . . So I haven't heard from him in, I want to say months, but it might even be at least a year. The last conversation I had with him, he was in really bad shape. His affect was really slowing down. I . . . spent three hours talking to him trying to convince him [not to commit suicide]. He didn't directly say, "I want to kill myself," but he said things like, "There is this mountain I need to climb and if I should fall off, then that is just the way it is." . . . And he did try to kill himself. I heard a few months back that he jumped onto a train track and someone pulled him out and he got into a fight with the person who pulled him out. That was a real sobering call that I got from my dad. You know when someone is being really self-destructive, but when you hear they tried to kill themselves, it changes everything. It was just . . . really a hard thing.

It was in speaking about his love for his brother that Jason offered some of his most provocative thoughts. The care and concern he feels toward Adam contrast with earlier descriptions of efforts to dissociate from his mother. When I asked about that difference Jason explained, "I don't think my brother has the same stalking mentality that my mother has." He continued by saying, "His situation is more touching to me [because] he has enough self-knowledge to be ashamed of his life. I think this is a big reason why he doesn't want to see me. He is ashamed of who he is. . . . He wants to be my big brother and here he is in mental institutions. I think it is the fact that I have a much deeper awareness of my brother's humanness that makes me more connected to him and more committed to him." These words helped me to understand one of Jason's earlier observations about his relationship with his mother. It was that he felt the full scope of his own life tragedy only in those few instances when his mother was able to act motherly. He put it this way:

My feelings for my brother are very different than my feelings for my mother. I think maybe it is because I have expectations of my parents. I mean, I am closer to my brother on some level than to my mother. It is very complex and it might not have as much to do with the fact that it is a sibling relationship than . . . with the fact that my brother has a level of self-awareness that my mother never had. And that might be why . . . when my mother demonstrates . . .

signs of selflessness towards me, that is when it really hurts. That is when I remember that my mother is my mother. She is acting like a mother and that is when the tragedy strikes me. That is when I get really sad and . . . when I really empathize with her. When she is stuck in the sort of the ego mode of her illness . . . it is really hard to empathize. She is so selfish in that world that it [only] makes me angry. . . . But when she does something which suggests to me that she cares about me and that she values what I value, then it hurts.

Aside from helping to explain the allocation of his own positive feelings between mother and brother, Jason's remarks illuminate one of the awful paradoxes of mental illness—the more care a mentally ill person needs, the less able are family members to provide it. The worse the illness, the harder it becomes for caregivers to remain compassionate. Throughout this book, respondents repeatedly distinguish between the person and the illness. When they feel negative emotions of anger, resentment, even hate, family members are quick to say that they continue to love the person kidnapped by the disease. To the degree that mental illness steals a person's essential humanity, makes the performance of conventional social roles impossible, and erodes their self-awareness, it expands emotional distance between caregiver and patient. When mentally ill people respond to medication and have periods of remission during which the "real" person reappears, caregivers more easily sustain both hope and commitment. However, the bonds of obligation become seriously frayed and sometimes broken altogether when a spouse, parent, child, or sibling seems permanently lost to mental illness.

Because of the trauma of his childhood and the continuing problems of his mother and brother, Jason devotes significant time to promoting his own healing. Perhaps it is because of the relentlessness of his mother's problems, despite the best efforts of psychiatrists, that Jason is so suspicious of the Western, medical model of mental illness. It is no great surprise that Jason has given a great deal of thought to the causes of mental illness. Through both experience and reading, he has become cynical about what he sees as "the narrow focus of the mental health industry." He explained his position by saying, "I'm pretty cynical because I haven't seen much help. I'm not cynical about the people who are trying to treat [the mentally ill]. I know there are good caring people who have their hearts in the right places and they really want to help my mother and brother, [but] I'm cynical about the emphasis on medication." Additional comments suggest that Jason has independently come to the sociological conclusion that comprehension of any illness experience requires looking at the intersection of body, mind, self, and society.[2] Here is how he thinks about the intersection of brain chemistry and cultural chemistry:

> I think people make a mistake when they equate mental illness with a chemical imbalance in the brain. For example, when you touch your hand to a hot stove, your brain chemistry is altered. That doesn't mean you need to adjust your brain chemistry, it means you need to get your hand off of the hot stove. So if the person's brain chemistry is out of balance it might be because there is something that isn't being addressed on some level, psychologically maybe. . . . It could [also] be lifestyle. It could be a person needs to become a priest and they are really working on Wall Street. . . . Or [it could be] a pathological life choice or a combination of bad life choices. . . . Or it could be . . . I think other societies have a place for a person . . . whose sensibility has been challenged to the degree that they are shaken up psychologically. . . . The Western model [of medicine] hasn't worked well enough. I mean, there are so many people who are suffering from one form of mental illness or another [that] something within our society is wrong.

Jason battles depression periodically, although, for reasons previously articulated, he has not relied on psychiatry for help. He did tell me, "I took Prozac very briefly. I didn't like it at all. I felt like [there was] this chemical straightjacket on my brain. It felt cold to me. I felt restrained." I asked Jason if he was afraid that he might someday become as ill as his mother or brother. He acknowledged "such a fear in the back of [his] mind," but worried more about his capacity to feel joy with abandon. He asks himself regularly, "Will I always be burdened by my life at some level? Will the burden itself become such a big part of me that I won't be able to separate that from my personality? . . . Will I always feel a sense of weight, of anxiety in my life [so that] I won't feel absolute joy? . . . You know . . . the kind of abandon that I wish I had in my life." Even though I found these to be eloquent expressions of his fears, Jason was not satisfied that they well enough captured his malaise. We pursued a different line of talk for a while, but then to clarify things, for both of us I imagine, he returned to a description of the pain associated with his particular "baggage":

> All I can do is describe sort of a sensation [I have]. . . . I am making a constant effort to make myself part of the world. . . . I am sort of emotionally grabbing the world on some level . . . because I have been separated from it. I think I have been so disoriented, so disconnected from myself and my surroundings that . . . I feel I have to make a constant effort to be connected. . . . I have had to constantly . . . make that effort to reconnect, whereas for people who have not been in as extreme a situation [as I have been], they are just naturally kind of connected. . . . Maybe I will always be on some level a little bit depressed, a little bit detached, a little bit alienated from myself, a little bit uncomfortable with myself and my life.

Most of the "children" I interviewed have maintained contact with their mentally ill mother or father. Their stories, however, are filled with uncertainty about what they continue to owe a parent whose illness literally deprived each of them of a normal childhood. Because of the particular circumstances of Jason's life, he has elected to divorce himself from any relationship with his mother. I suspect that other children of mentally ill parents would not judge Jason harshly for his choice. They would understand that children do not own their parents everything. They would also understand that after reasonable efforts to save a parent have failed, it becomes a person's primary obligation to save themselves.

Am I My Brother's Keeper?

Angie's brother died about four years before we spoke. During the last year of his life Paul's health had badly deteriorated and he was constantly in and out of the hospital. His life ended on a highway where he was struck down by a tractor trailer. Although the coroner ruled it a suicide, Angie doubted that her brother had planned to kill himself. At the time of the accident, she told me, "he was totally out of it, totally irrational." Before the accident, they later learned, he had been running along the highway, trying to stop people to ask for help "because he thought he was being chased by helicopters and the police." At age thirty-seven, Angie was still piecing together the nature of her older brother's (by three years) illness, the circumstances of their growing up, why it took her so long to understand his suffering, her distinctive role as a sibling, the continuing impact of her family's history on her relationships and life aspirations, and the guilt she still feels about Paul's death.

For the past ten years Angie had been working in Boston as an office manager in the financial industry. She explained that because her parents and brother had lived in Virginia, "I wasn't exposed to my brother on a daily basis . . . so it's a little harder to comprehend things when you're not spending a lot of time with him. . . . You only see glimpses of it. . . . It wasn't until I was getting close to thirty that I saw him at a really bad stage. It was obvious that he was totally hallucinogenic and . . . that's when I actually *got it*." Of course, Angie understood well before turning thirty that her brother was schizophrenic, but, as a sibling, did not quite appreciate what his illness meant. "A lot of times mental illness is a hard thing to understand," Angie told me. "I knew my brother was ill," she continued, "but I always thought that he used it to manipulate people. . . . I mean, my brother was demanding as a teenager and . . . my mother used to get upset with me when he was ill because I'd get

mad at him. . . . You know, like any brother and sister we'd fight."
By age thirty, however, she understood the severity of Paul's illness
and the huge toll it exacted from her parents. It was only then that
the emotional struggle to figure out her obligations to Paul and her
aging parents truly began.

Even though she grew up in a home dominated by mental illness,
Angie did not remember her childhood explicitly in illness terms.
Before her brother began to exhibit symptoms in his late teens, she
had to negotiate around a father whom she later learned was mentally ill. As a child she knew only that her father "was taking medications and a lot of times his tongue would swell and he couldn't
talk, and things like that." She was enough aware of her dad's difficulties to be embarrassed when friends thought he was drunk.
Although Angie would explain that her father was on medications,
she didn't know exactly why he was obliged to take them. As I
frequently heard, parents conspired to insulate a healthy child from
family illness. "My mother never really explained . . . what was going on. Unless someone sits you down and explains to you, you
don't really know. . . . I think that for the most part my mother
reacted like everything was normal. . . . [My father] sat in the living
room all by himself and we could hear him talking to himself . . .
but I never felt comfortable to say, 'What's wrong?' "

Miraculously, Angie's father experienced a remission and was
able to resume a normal work life. However, just as her father
became healthy, Paul began to deteriorate. By her teenage years,
Angie finally learned that Paul suffered from schizophrenia. She
also learned that she was expected to keep his illness a family secret.
"There were a lot of secrets," she said, "and I think that because
of my parents' age and generation they felt . . . ashamed. . . . For the
longest time, my mother used to say, 'Now, don't say anything if
you run into your friends, don't say anything about your brother.' "
Even though she comprehended that Paul was sick, she still responded to him more primarily as a brother who was "just being
his usual self, being pushy and lazy and getting out of work like he
always did when he was a teenager. . . . I never really knew what

was going on.... I thought a lot of it was just his personality."
Even later, Angie recalled, she treated her brother's symptoms far
more lightly than could her parents. She recounted how, after
having left home, she would joke with Paul about his delusions
during her periodic visits:

> I know my brother had the same thing [as my father].... I used to
> go on walks with him and I'd say something to him and he wouldn't
> respond. He had a good sense of humor and so I said to him, "Paul,
> the voices, they get to talk to you all the time. I don't see you very
> often. Tell them to shut up and talk to me!" [said while laughing].
> And it was funny. Though he was totally preoccupied before, he
> heard that, and he said, "Okay, I'm sorry," and he started laughing.
> ... It got to the point that he wasn't able to hold down a job, so he
> basically had to live with my parents. He was so paranoid that people
> were listening outside his window that they had to get air condi-
> tioning because he would not let them open the windows in the
> summer. So, it's amazing what families do to accommodate. But I'd
> go home and visit and I'd open the window because I don't like air
> conditioning and he'd get so upset with me. Finally, I'd say, "What
> do you have to say that somebody is going to want to hear?" [laugh-
> ing]. He wouldn't be mad or anything. He'd say, "I know I'm not
> being rational and I know you think I'm being ridiculous, but I can't
> help it."

Although physically removed from the day-to-day turmoil connected with Paul's illness, much of Angie's life was still significantly
bounded by her difficult family history. To tell or not to tell friends
about mental illness at home is typically an emotionally charged
question for healthy family members. In this matter, Angie has
largely chosen to rebel against the legacy of secrecy about Paul's
and her father's mental illness. "I told people that my brother was
schizophrenic, which my parents don't like. When they come to
visit, they'd be like, 'Did you tell them [friends]?' I'd say, 'No, I
didn't,' but I had. I didn't feel the need to hide it, but I understand

why other people do, because there are a lot of misconceptions [about mental illness]." To illustrate, she described having once told a friend that her brother was schizophrenic and he replied, "I'm sorry your brother is crazy." Trying to educate him, she responded, "Paul is not crazy, he's schizophrenic. I don't think you understand. You don't know what schizophrenia is." She went on to explain, "My brother is very rational in many ways. It's just in certain areas he's not rational. . . . He does my mother's investing and he's great at it."

Despite her commitment to truth-telling with friends, she did acknowledge that the problem of disclosure remains complicated. Angie admits that she would like to remarry and have children. As much as she would like to be up-front with boyfriends about her family difficulties, decisions about the timing of such news are delicate. Here's how she described the dilemma surrounding truth-telling: "You're kind of damned if you do, damned if you don't. . . . When I date people, I always think, 'Now, how am I going to tell them?' Before my brother passed away, I was like, 'How do you bring up the fact that your brother's schizophrenic and . . . it runs in your family?' [slight laugh] I mean, how *do* you bring that up?"

In one case, Angie dated a man for a year and a half without discussing mental illness, all the while burdened by the feelings of dishonesty occasioned by silence. At the time of our interview, she was dating a man whose mother had been diagnosed with manic-depressive illness. Understanding the irony of her own attitude, she described this relationship as unusual because "I've always avoided people from dysfunctional families. I've had enough of it! [laughing]. I don't want to take on any more." Then, with a hint of sadness, she said, "The fact of the matter is I'm thirty-seven and I'm realistic. Who's really going to want to marry into the genes I have?" Her comment prompted me to pose a difficult question. I asked Angie, "Do you feel somehow tainted or damaged?" At first, she simply said, "Yeah." Then she went on to say:

> Well, not damaged. I've said to my friends, I have something that I
> have to deal with, not as a result of anything I've done, but because

of my family history. And, it's not an easy thing to deal with. Mental illness is not a fun subject and a lot of people don't understand it. And it's kind of like, "Okay this is something that I have to deal with. It's not anything that I have control over. . . . It's just something that I've come to deal with. I've come to accept it. I don't think I really resent it. . . . I think it's made me more sensitive. . . . [But] love is not blind when you get older. I think there's a very rational side to it. . . . Well, my brother and I had this conversation too. He said, "Angie, if you ever get married again you shouldn't have kids." It is something [to think about]. I would never want anybody to go through what my brother went through.

It is a simple truth of sociology that each of us sees the world differently depending on where we stand in it. Angie understood that for many years she saw her brother very differently from how her parents did because "siblings see brothers and sisters differently than other people do." As you have seen, the sibling vantage point, combined with her parents' secrecy, made it difficult for Angie to realize the severity of her brother's problems. As all of us move through the life course, however, we begin to see people and events from fresh angles. As Angie expressed it, "It wasn't until our late twenties [or] early thirties that I saw Paul as an adult." When they were kids, Paul was a loner who liked reading and growing orchids, unusual hobbies to an outgoing, athletic sister who was far more interested in boys than books. After a failed marriage and relocation to Boston, Angie "started reading a lot more" and "just kind of grew and matured" in a way that caused her to better appreciate Paul's interests.

By her early thirties, Angie also saw her parents differently. Now, well into their sixties, she could more clearly notice how Paul's illness was "really wearing on them." As they aged, Paul's illness picked up a distressing momentum, requiring multiple hospitalizations. "There were times," Angie reported, "that I would go down and visit and he was so bad that they hadn't let my parents see him." She only got to see him after announcing, "I'm his sister from out of town, could you make an exception?" When he did come home, somebody always had to be with Paul. Angie's dilemma was compounded when her mother began to hint that she ought to return home to help. She described her feelings by saying, "They [parents] had no breaks and I think my family wanted me to move home, but to be perfectly honest I didn't want to move back. . . . I didn't want to deal with all the dysfunction." Questions about returning home prompted Angie to talk volubly about her "struggle." I expect that any adult siblings of mentally ill brothers and sisters reading this account will understand the emotional confusion and deep ambivalence Angie felt when she said:

> It's kind of hard to put [my feelings] into words. I mean I love my parents dearly and I love my brother, and I think you're raised to know what's right and wrong. And I do feel like your family comes first. But by the same token, how much . . . is realistic for a sibling to give up? Are you supposed to give up your life? And [give up] your career? I mean, [do you give up] your hopes? I was divorced. Should I have to give up the possibility of getting remarried because my brother is ill? But is it fair for my parents, in their sixties, to have to deal with this after they're retired? I mean, my father retired at fifty-five and was looking forward to traveling and doing other things. And you know, they had worked all their lives and now they had to take care of my brother. That didn't seem fair. And it's like where do you draw the line? Just where do you draw the line? Do you do what's right for your family and just do it unselfishly? It's a hard thing. It's easy to say, "Yeah, I'd do anything for my family" until you really have to, until you are faced with it.

Angie talked with great intensity about her ongoing efforts to answer the question "Am I entitled to live my own life?" Long after the fact of Paul's death—perhaps because of his death—Angie was still persuading herself that she made appropriate moral choices. During the course of our conversation she repeatedly used the words *struggle* and *guilt*. Several times, when expressing her distress at the prospect of returning to her parents' home, she said, virtually as a kind of apology to me, "I'm just trying to be very honest." Her decisions at the time were complicated by her mother's expectations. Although her father told her privately, "You have your own life to live; this is your mother's and my problem to deal with," she knew her mother did not share that perspective. She explained, "I couldn't talk to my mother about it because she had this attitude like, 'That's your . . . brother and you should do everything you possibly can.' "

During the hour or so that Angie talked about the distress surrounding obligations, she made explicit the terms of her internal debate. "Should I give up having a life, like my parents did, to help my brother who was getting progressively worse? You go back and forth. There is no clear answer." Returning home helped to clarify things because, she told me, "I'd go down there and I'd be exhausted, but my mother would put up with my brother. . . . It wore on my nerves. I just couldn't imagine [being there]." Sometimes during those visits Angie would raise alternatives to her brother's remaining at home, telling her parents, "Maybe it would be helpful if Paul were in a halfway house. . . . You've kept him here and you've tried to help him, but he's not getting any better. He's getting worse." However, these conversations were short-lived since her mother dismissed the ideas without discussion. Realizing that changes at home were unlikely, Angie had to find reasons why it would, in fact, be best if she did not return home. These are some of the things she told me and, I presume, over and over, herself:

I thought, "Well maybe if I brought him up here [Boston], I could supervise him," but I was just making ends meet. [If I had the money] I would have brought him up here in a heartbeat. It would have been good for my parents and good for him. If I had more money and more resources available to me I would have done some other things to help my brother. [But without money] your hands are kind of tied.

↩

I guess my mother and I are just different.... Maybe she's more unselfish than I am. She would do whatever had to be done, [whereas] I think sometimes you have to be a bit more logical.

↜

If I get married and have children ... it's not fair to subject them to [Paul's illness]. I don't think that's fair to do to children. It's not their burden to bear. Is it fair to disrupt several families because of one person? I mean, you would really disrupt the person you marry and in a sense his family is really married into it. How much is it fair to disrupt for one person?

You already know that during the course of considering what was practical, fair, and moral to do, Paul died. Of course, had all the dilemmas associated with Paul's illness disappeared with his passing, Angie would likely never have responded to the newspaper advertisement that led to our meeting. I hope that our conversation gave her yet another chance to sort out the complexities of a sister's obligations both to her brother and her parents. However, as our conversation turned to the aftermath of Paul's death, it was clear that everyone's suffering continues, especially Angie's mother's. As though I needed to have it yet again affirmed, she told me, "My mother is an extremely compassionate person.... She has a lot of guilt. She says, 'I didn't do enough. I should have done this or I should have done that.' And I said, 'You took care of him for years and years and years. You never gave up trying to get him help, looking for a cure.'" This line of conversation led to yet another hesitant admission from Angie. Here's how our talk proceeded:

Well, emotions aren't rational, by definition. Emotions are beyond reason.

That's true ... and maybe I shouldn't say this, but my mother still wishes my brother was alive. And I said to her, "The last year Paul was alive he was really ill. And he used to say, 'All I want for me is peace.' He explained to me, 'I never have peace.' "

This is your brother speaking?

Yeah, he said, "I hear voices constantly and it doesn't stop at night; it doesn't stop all day long."

It's an unimaginable thing.

Yeah and he said, "You can't imagine." I said, "I don't know how you deal with it." And he said, "You have no peace. All I want is peace." And . . . the last couple years [of his life], he had a lot of other health problems as a result [of his illness]. I mean the medications take a toll on your body and because he'd been taking them for, you know, over ten years, they really took a toll. I mean he was having trouble with his stomach and all kinds of other things. And he's like, "I have no peace. My mind is constantly going. I can't even sleep at night. It never shuts off. . . . All I really want is some peace. I want peace of mind." And so, I get angry with my mother sometimes because all he ever wanted was some peace, and now he has peace. And [she] wants him to be here suffering, rather than letting him have his peace. He hasn't had peace in ten years. . . . I say let him rest in peace.

You might think from these sentiments that Angie is herself free of guilt about Paul's difficult life and death. In fact, she continued to feel guilty about all those times during their childhood years when she was impatient, lost her temper, or simply treated him like any brother who annoys a sister. With the perspective that history always provides, Angie realized that she simply didn't understand his illness. Now, with Paul gone, she expressed amazement about his own patience in the face of her incomprehension. Toward the very end of our conversation, Angie described yet another source of guilt. Reminiscent of the warning to be careful what you wish for since you might get it, Angie talked about the guilt that can arise when prayers are answered. This is how she explained feeling guilty about having prayed for the "wrong" thing:

> Even as a teenager I had trouble with all the conflict ... going on in the family. ... I would always say to my brother [that] when I went to church I prayed for him. And ... I've said to one of my friends [who is] somewhat religious, "I used to always pray for my brother to get peace of mind, for him to get peace of mind." When he was in his accident, I came back and I was very upset and she said "What's the matter?" and I said, "I feel guilty. I prayed for the wrong thing. I prayed for him to have peace of mind. I should have prayed for him to get better." I feel guilty because I prayed for the wrong thing.

More understandable to me was Angie's addendum that "I [also] kind of feel guilty because I am the surviving sibling." When she revealed this last source of guilt to her father, he replied, "That's funny because your mother said almost the same thing to me." With the slightly self-conscious laugh that accompanied a number of difficult truths throughout our interview, Angie concluded, "I guess I'm more like my mother than I wanted to think."

In Sickness and in Health

Work, marriage, and motherhood were persistent themes in the conversations among the six women in Gail's college sorority. Raised in Charlotte, North Carolina, Gail elected to attend a large southern university even though she would be one of only about 200 Jewish students on the campus. Remarkably, all six sorority sisters fell in love during their college years and decided to collectively plan the timing of their respective weddings. Gail explained how "all six of us got married the same summer and we planned it out perfectly." Now, five years later Gail could compare college fantasies with current realities. For those among the six still living in the South, with children and conventional careers, life is pretty much as they pictured in college. Although one friend is now divorced, none of the women have experienced anything like the unexpected turmoil in Gail's life. Shortly after their first anniversary, Jeff suffered a manic episode. Now, after four years of dealing with a chronically depressed and often suicidal husband, Gail is surely correct that, compared to her college friends, "she and Jeff have experienced much more in life than they have, than they [likely] ever will."

Jeff had already survived a personal tragedy well before meeting Gail. As an outstanding high school football player, "one of the two best in the state his senior year," he had been wooed by several colleges. Shortly after choosing the college where his dad had played ball, Jeff accidentally fell four stories over a balcony "too short for such a tall man." Although "they actually didn't think he was going to live after the accident," Jeff remarkably entered college that same year "on crutches with all those rods in his hands and legs." By the end of his sophomore year, still nurturing dreams of a professional football career, he tried once again to play. The combination of pain and physical limitations crushed, with distressing finality, any hopes for an athletic career. As Gail recalled, "That was when he first started having all of his emotional problems, so everyone linked it to that." She now realizes that Jeff's emotional difficulties arise more primarily from manic-depressive illness, although she has observed, among other patterns, that he "becomes severely depressed every time football season comes around."

One of the things that worried Gail shortly after meeting him was Jeff's anger. On occasion she saw signs of violence when he drank with buddies, something that she largely "wrote off . . . as just the regular behavior [of] . . . a bunch of drunk fraternity guys." She remembered that "he never hit anybody, but he would sometimes hit a wall or scream and curse, things like that." They talked about it at Gail's insistence so that he would know that "[violence] was something I wouldn't accept," that if "anything ever happened to me physically . . . I was out the door. [I said that] while we were still dating." Based on her own training as a clinical social worker, Jeff's behaviors over several years, and his eventual diagnosis, Gail now better understands his anger as the product of illness. She told me:

> He has rage the size of a city inside this one man's body. I would be afraid to be around if it ever came out . . . and I have told him that. The little violence that I saw when he used to drink . . . I see every once in a while when he gets pushed over the edge. One time a car cut me off. He jumped out of the car like he was going to do something and, of course, the people were gone and I was like, "Get back in the car!" When he got back in he was just trembling . . . [with] that kind of rage.

As I heard many times previously, it was a concrete incident that forced Gail to realize that her husband's problems and erratic behaviors were caused by mental illness. I asked her to describe the first moment she knew that something was desperately wrong with her husband. She recounted a series of events that led to his psychotic breakdown barely a year after they married. A psychiatrist had prescribed Prozac for Jeff three or four weeks before his decomposition. Jeff had also just spent several days tending, with little sleep, to Gail's hospitalized father who had been badly injured in an automobile accident. When Jeff finally came home, Gail left to maintain the hospital vigil. On arriving there, she received a panicky call from a younger brother demanding that she return home immediately. Jeff was acting very strangely. Gail interrupted the narrative to hypothesize that the combination of Prozac, sleep deprivation, and family stress had propelled Jeff into mania. The incident unfolded this way:

> The next thing I know, while I am talking to him, he climbs out on the roof. I would say the first moment I knew . . . that he had mental illness was when he was on my roof. That was just a few years ago

and he was actually having a hallucination. He thought that I had cops there and I didn't yet. It was blowing my mind. He kept saying, "Get the cops out. Get the cops out." And I am going, "Cut this out!"

It must be an incredible moment to absorb the fact that this is a deranged person up there.

Yeah, that is exactly what happened. . . . It was when he was up on the roof and then I couldn't get him down and I said [to myself], "I don't know what he would do if he came down." I was thinking, "He could get a knife out of the kitchen." I was thinking the worst, of course, because that is how frightened I got. I felt like "this is a crazy man on the roof. How the hell did he get on the roof?" I don't even know how he got up there. We don't have a house that it was easy to just jump on the roof. So . . . he had so much adrenaline going that he found some way to climb up the gutter. . . . At one o'clock in the morning, I called my best friend from social work school in another city to ask her what to do. Then I called the crisis center [where] I had volunteered . . . and they were like, "Gail, call the police, what are you talking about!" But I was thinking, "Oh no, we can deal with it. We can deal with it." And then finally I said, "No, I have to call 911."

As a social worker, if you had been the recipient of the call, you probably would have advised calling the police right away.

Oh, immediately I would have known what to do. Sure, definitely, but I was thinking of all the other people. I was thinking, "Oh my God, what do I do with my little brother?" I was thinking my mom and my sister are at the hospital with my father. I was thinking, you know, "How the hell are we going to deal with it?" All I kept thinking was, "If I could just get him inside, get him medicine to go to sleep, he'll be okay." But the scary thing when [someone] goes crazy [is that] you can't do anything. . . . They did have to heavily sedate

him once they got him to the hospital. Yeah, so that was the first
time I really knew that he had something wrong with him.

The last four years of their marriage have been dominated by
Jeff's illness. Shortly into our conversation, Gail tried to explain her
ongoing commitment to her spouse, as well as the conditions under
which she might have to leave him. My routine question about
religious affiliation led to expansive talk about the links among her
spiritual beliefs, family values, and personal commitments. Because
of her strong attachment to Judaism, Gail did not envision mar-
rying a non-Jew before meeting Jeff. After marriage, Jeff actually
began the process of conversion to Judaism. Although illness interrupted his life so often that he never officially completed the conversion, she explained that "when we meet people we tell them that
we are Jewish because there is no sense in trying to explain the
whole story." She went on to say:

> I think the times when Jeff and I have lived the most normal, happy
> parts of our lives were when we were both actively practicing our
> religion, when we were going to synagogue every week. Like . . . right
> now, every Friday night we have a Shabbot dinner by ourselves . . .
> those kind of things.[3] We call my family because we are not there
> with them and some of those traditions bring out and help to carry
> on other values . . . like commitment to one another. . . . When you
> celebrate the traditions like the Shabbot dinner . . . it definitely brings
> back the sense of dedication to a commitment. You can't give up!
> . . . [Among] Jewish values is the dependability of family for every-
> thing . . . you know, sustaining each other and sticking together.

Although Gail's commitment to Jeff and to their marriage
seemed strong at the time of our conversation, she did admit that
she sometimes wonders whether she can sustain the relationship.
At one point she acknowledged, "I'd be lying to you if I said I
haven't been emotionally scarred from his illness because I'm sure
that I have." Later, she described how, shortly after moving to Bos-

ton to pursue a Ph.D. in a prestigious graduate program, Jeff fell
into "one of his suicidal states and I thought, 'I'm never going to
be able to do this [graduate school] with him like this.' " "There
are times," she continued, "when I feel like, 'God, maybe my life
would be better off if I wasn't with him.' " It does not help matters
that Jeff himself urges her to leave the marriage when he is most
suicidal. Indeed, during the three hours we spent together, Gail
expressed the greatest distress about Jeff's suicide talk. Hearing that
he did not want to live hurt deeply because it seemed a denial of the
redemptive power of their love. Describing a recent episode, Gail
said, "He was incredibly suicidal and I don't know how long I can
live with someone [like that]." She told me that if Jeff actually did
commit suicide, her response wouldn't be "Oh he was so sick." It
would be, "God damned, he didn't love me enough to stay with me."

As Gail detailed her joint marital and illness history with Jeff, I
was once again impressed by how powerfully love catalyzes commitment. She told me that "over the past two years I've had eight
million people say to me, 'Why are you staying with him?' " Her
response? "Because we do have a truly sincere love for each other
and I would have to say that if that went away it would make me
question things a lot more." Clearly, it would be impossible to
sustain their marriage without love. However, listening to Gail I
sensed that, over the long haul, love might not be enough. At one
point, I remarked that she seemed to have a sort of "additive"
model of injury to their relationship. She agreed that each of the
traumas, hurts, disappointments, and compromises generated by
Jeff's illness chips away at the solidity of their life together. Four
years after the onset of his illness, Gail is still struggling to "find
[her] role as a professional, married woman who may have to be
the sole supporter of her family and yet still be a wife and not a
mother—because when he is really sick I would describe my behavior [toward him] as mother-like." Having read this far in the
book, you should not be surprised by the multiple ways Jeff's mental illness compromises the discovery of such a role.

My work as an interviewer is premised on the notion that words, as much as eyes, are a window into souls and minds. Throughout our talk Gail used the language of accommodation, compromise, modification, adjustment, and adaptation to describe her response to Jeff's illness. In order to make the right adjustments in her own behavior and their joint lifestyle, Gail has become exquisitely tuned into the subtleties of Jeff's moods and behaviors. Like a meteorologist who must be on the lookout for disturbing weather patterns long before they actually arrive on the scene, Gail has become expert at reading signs of impending difficulty so that illness storms might be avoided. For instance, knowing that Jeff "gets really really upset about the fact that we owe money for medical bills . . . I take it all on myself. . . . I'm the one who calls everybody to say that we are late on the bills. . . . If I tell him that we don't have a lot of money this week . . . he would freak out [and] stop eating." Gail often cajoles Jeff into going to bed or waking at certain times because she knows that "if he gets off kilter it is going to take him weeks to get back to a regular schedule." In a variety of similar ways, Gail must be careful to avoid behaviors and situations that "would throw [Jeff's] illness into high gear."

Although Gail continues to learn about the various signals that allow her to forestall trouble, her task is, in fact, quite like weather prediction in the Northeast, where I live. New Englanders joke that if you don't like the weather, just hang around a bit because it changes so abruptly and unpredictably. Despite her best efforts to head off illness episodes, Gail never knows just when Jeff is going to "flip." She explained that "there is a part of me that thinks, 'Oh, if I don't do this or that . . . he's going to flip over the edge, because he has really quick cycles.'" While she believes that she will eventually "know enough of [Jeff's] patterns to be able to live more comfortably than I am now," Gail admits to "walking on eggshells." It must greatly erode the quality of daily life when a spouse doesn't know "if it's okay to talk, to bring up subjects," when "there are a lot of things that bring out [the illness] that I . . . don't know [will]." Even the most routine features of everyday life cannot be taken for granted when a family member is mentally ill.[4] Gail put it this way:

It makes us think harder about everything . . . [about] the things that we take for granted in life, I guess. [For example], we take for granted that a vacation is a good thing, but with someone like Jeff riding on an airplane with a bunch of people who might be rude . . . and [then] waiting a lot . . . really has a very yucky impact on him. So sometimes taking a vacation is not a fun thing for us. So we choose not to sometimes. Things that other people just don't even think about. . . . I think [mental illness] makes you more aware of your surroundings and what you are willing to put yourself into. . . . Some people would say that this is really bad that it makes us always think about what we are going to do "if." You know, [they say], "Why do you always worry about the ifs?" But we need to know what we would do if something occurred. . . . I don't think that that is such a bad thing, knowing our past history.

Like nearly all caregivers, Gail sometimes wonders whether her husband uses his illness to manipulate her. He certainly succeeds in making her feel guilty "for doing things without him, for being at work too much, for things like that." As further illustration, she told me that even getting to our interview posed a slight problem. "There was a little bit of 'Oh don't leave me' going on when I left." Although Gail told me that deciding whether to accommodate Jeff's wishes is "something I deal with on a daily basis," she is less likely to capitulate to her husband's ongoing demands now that she "realize[s] the dynamics of the illness." "Earlier," she told me, "I would do just about anything he wanted. He would wake me up at four o'clock in the morning and say, 'I really need to go get something to eat.' Whereas now I would be like, 'Sorry buster, there is something in the fridge.' "

Some accommodations are more easily made than others. Although an ill person's daily, unremitting demands significantly erode attachments, it is still one thing to adjust bedtimes and quite another to modify career aspirations. The elements of mental illness most threatening to Gail's marriage are those that compromise her largest life hopes and aspirations. Five years into a marriage significantly defined by mental illness, Gail must contend with reframing her life plans. Whatever life bumps her sorority sisters might have absorbed, they were still largely pursuing the dreams they shared in college. With only slight detours, they are still building families and careers essentially on schedule.

As several social scientists[5] have observed, a critical aspect of the "normal" aging experience in any society is not just doing things in the right sequence but, equally important, doing them at the proper time. Although age-related norms are subject to change and vary by social class, studies of middle-class groups show high agreement about the "appropriate" age for moving through major points in the life course—finishing school, marriage, settling into a career, having children, becoming grandparents, and retiring.[6] At age twenty-eight, Gail was beginning to feel more acutely the dislocation of being "off time." She was already significantly far enough from the normal time track to realize the widening distance between the anticipation of her life and its actuality. These are some of her reflections on the more painful accommodations required to reconstruct an entire life blueprint:

> I didn't think that I'd be the sole [family] earner. In my mind now I have to know that I could be the sole earner forever. . . . I mean, I can do it [because] I never wanted to be . . . just a housewife. . . . I always knew I wanted to work when we met. [So], when we got married the things that would go through my mind were, "Okay, when am I going to have kids [and] will I still be able to work and do these kinds of things?" So, right now . . . that has totally changed and I have to get this [Ph.D.] degree in order to get a decent job that could support us, and if we have a family could also support our family. [Having a child] is another whole complicated thing that I sometimes don't even deal with because I don't know if that is even a possibility any more. [That] is definitely a disappointment to me. . . . My uncle has bipolar illness that I was never told about until about a year ago. . . . So [there is] the fear that [because of] Jeff's direct genetics and my indirect genetics we might have a child who would be really ill.

Following these comments, I asked Gail just how hard it has been to revise downward some of her aspirations and she replied:

> I guess I'm okay with it but . . . I have tons of anger, not really to him—sometimes to him—but more to, you know, "Why me?" Why did this happen to me? Why did my husband happen to be the one who got ill? Because when we got married, we were the perfect little couple. . . . So, yes, I've had to revise a lot. . . . I can't think that far in advance any more. That is probably the biggest thing that has changed in my life because I used to be a planner, all the time planning—ten years ahead. . . . With an illness like this that runs in cycles . . . I just think it's too much to put on yourself to expect things when you don't know what's going to happen.

In Chapter 3, "Managing Emotions," I relied heavily on a book by the sociologist Arlie Russell Hochschild entitled *The Managed Heart*.[7] Exploring America's transition from a production- to a service-oriented economy, the book shows that service occupations require workers to "manage their hearts" by suppressing their true feelings. Such work, Hochschild argues, produces a kind of emotional alienation just as powerful and destructive as the sort of alienation produced by the nineteenth-century factory system described by Karl Marx.[8]

When Gail described efforts to mute "tons of anger," it seemed apparent that Hochschild's ideas easily extend to caregiving as a form of service work. Because family caregivers must manage their hearts, they no doubt feel a type of emotional alienation. Unlike the airline stewardesses studied by Hochschild who have no genuine commitment to the passengers they serve, the emotional alienation felt by spouses like Gail is no doubt blunted by honest love. Nevertheless, the obligation to give up cherished life plans because of another person's illness inevitably creates a deep disjunction between inner feelings and outward expressions of care. At a certain point, even love is not enough to contain feelings of anger and disappointment.

> I have real good denial skills in that I can gloss over things and make like everything is okay on the outside and then come home and crash. Maybe not even crash, but just have it build up inside. I know that that is a technique that I have used all of my life and especially with him, but over the past two years it's been harder to do.... He has seen me have to take incompletes in classes and I know that he has had terrible guilt over that.... I definitely still do have anger that I might have to take a class over ... so what do you do? I am really angry. I am pissed off.... He has a lot of guilt because he feels like he's stopped me from a lot of things. Well, *he has*! I can't play like he hasn't anymore.

Before we left each other, my conversation with Gail touched on a number of familiar issues. Even though she has training in social work, Gail complained bitterly at several points about the infuriating difficulty in navigating a hopelessly complex mental health system. Coupled with insurance horror stories, Gail told of hospital stays that "basically just kept [Jeff] alive" and left him with a tainted identity. Our talk also touched on her efforts to educate parents and friends about Jeff's illness so that she can tell the truth when they ask how things are going. Honest accounts about her own well-being would, unfortunately, also require Gail to describe her own treatment for depression. "My bouts of depression," Gail explained, "have been when he gets really sick and then starts to get better ... because, of course, I'd be a little off the burner."

Although Jeff pessimistically characterizes his as a terminal illness that will eventually kill him one way or another, Gail nevertheless holds onto her optimism. After enduring the distressing side effects and eventual failure of various drug therapies, Jeff has been responsive to electroconvulsive (ECT) treatments. Once he finally "hooked up with a doctor who is a real pain in the ass to insurance people," Jeff received a series of twelve ECT sessions. While hardly a cure, Gail could say at the time of our interview that, as a result of the ECT therapy, "We are living a seminormal life. If you didn't know that he had bipolar illness . . . you wouldn't know anything was any different. If you didn't ask him what he did for a living or anything like that, you would think he was just a regular guy. When we go out to a restaurant people think we are just regular people." To approximate the life of "regular" people is no small triumph for folks like Gail and Jeff. Several weeks before writing these pages I spoke with Gail and was happy to learn that, after another round of ECT, Jeff continues to do well.

One can only guess about the likelihood of any marriage succeeding, much less one hobbled by mental illness. I hope that I am right in predicting that Gail and Jeff will stay together. Jeff is fortunate to have a partner who loves him deeply, who is resolute in her determination to help, who embraces a value system that prizes commitments, and whose natural inclination is to be optimistic. Were these the only positive things I could say about their relationship I might not be so sanguine about its longevity. There is one additional ingredient that is absolutely necessary if a marriage weighted down by mental illness is to survive. Caregiving spouses must truly incorporate two fundamental ideas into their thinking and be guided by them in their daily lives. The first is that that they cannot solve the problem. The second is that they must somehow preserve the integrity of their own life and identity. Toward the end of our time together Gail described this critical shift in her thinking:

> You must realize that you still have to have your own life. . . . I have to have me in order to be able to live with him. You know, people say you have to be able to help yourself to help someone else. . . . I think that is part of why we can stay together, at least for now. I am me and I do have my own life and my own goals and expectations and they are not completely . . . enmeshed in his illness. I think

if I stayed buried by it all of the time . . . things would get bad
enough for me to need to leave.

Like most essential truths, there is a simplicity to Gail's prescription for maintaining her marriage and her commitment to Jeff. I hope she succeeds in constructing a life consistent with the wisdom of her own words, in both good times and bad.

In his 1951 masterpiece *Rashomon*, the Japanese filmmaker Akiro Kurosawa told a story of four witnesses to a violent rape and murder. As the film depicts the crime from each character's point of view, we realize how dramatically different the same event can be seen, depending on one's relationship to it. *Rashomon* illustrates the relativity of truth and the inevitable subjectivity that shapes both perception and experience. Through the cases studies offered in this chapter and others presented earlier, you have seen that mental illness has widely varying effects on the lives of parents, children, siblings, and spouses. Just days before writing these words, I heard a similar point made by a young woman in the Wednesday night Family and Friends group. Like many children growing up with a sick parent, she explained that she could not even identify her mother's problem as mental illness until she was seventeen. After trying to capture the distinctiveness of her experience as a "child," she ended with the simple but profound thought that, compared with the parents, siblings, and spouses in the group, hers was just "another way of learning" about mental illness.

The woman's astute comment suggests that family members follow fundamentally different routes in learning exactly how mental illness affects a loved one and, ultimately, their own life. Like the four characters in *Rashomon*, parents, children, siblings, and spouses have different perceptions and experiences on *everything* affecting the life of a family. In large part, these differences arise from the distinctive roles each performs in the family's emotional, economic, and practical division of labor. To be a parent, for example, means to have a certain kind of relationship with children. As Jason put it earlier, "It is terrifying to a child when the parent needs to be nurtured. I mean, when you are eight, nine, ten, eleven years old it is terrifying to a child to have your parent be helpless. . . . This is not the 'right role.' " Just as there are "right" roles between parents and children, so are there right roles that govern the relationships of siblings, spouses, and children. Occupying different locations within the ecology of the family ensures that each family member will have a "different way of learning" about mental illness.

The notion of "right roles" also implies general cultural guidelines that dictate the moral obligations among family members when one of them requires care. There appears to be a "hierarchy of obligations" when it comes to determining who should be most centrally involved in a family member's care.[9] While we clearly share common ideas about the "proper thing to do" when a mother, father, sister, brother, son, or daughter becomes ill, the stories offered in this chapter also show that the strength of kinship ties varies from family to family and that the distribution of care is always negotiated in terms of particular family contingencies. Jason and Angie, especially, described painful ambivalence as they tried to decide the extent of their family responsibilities. Their accounts remind us that obligations are always the product of ongoing interpretations within particular contexts. Nevertheless, the interview materials presented in the first four chapters suggest these genealogical rules as normally determining the distribution of care within kinship networks.

- We have greater obligations to those in our immediate families than to members of our extended families.
- The strongest caregiving ties within families are between spouses and between parents and their immature children.
- Spouses must rely on each other for care before expecting the help of children.

- Obligations to ill children are the most powerful and enduring of all obligations.
- Duties toward one's parents and children are much stronger than toward brothers and sisters.
- Parents have diminished claims on the support of their children once they have married.
- Parental claims for support are further weakened once their children have children of their own.

The stories told in this chapter help us to understand how caregivers' perspectives are influenced by their place in the family. Parents, spouses, children, and siblings feel, more or less intensely, the obligation to care. Each has a different calculus defining what they owe others and what their obligations are to themselves. There is, however, an even more powerful and encompassing regularity that shapes the hierarchy of family obligations. Whenever both men and women are potential caregivers, women nearly always take on more responsibility. Mothers are normally more deeply invested in caring for children than their husbands. When children are old enough to care for ill parents, daughters are ordinarily expected to be more involved in caring than sons. When an ill person has both brothers and sisters, the sisters typically take the caregiving lead. No cultural factor has greater weight or sheer force in determining caregiving roles than gender. By now, you have already heard some of my thinking on why this is so. I will, though, return to this critical matter in the remaining chapters, especially in Chapter 7.

The first four chapters suggest another set of questions that fundamentally shape the perspectives and behaviors of caregivers. In the context of tremendous uncertainty, family members inevitably assess the causes of mental illness, the likelihood of its ever being cured, and their own role in trying, at the least, to control it. Ideas about cause, cure, and control define the boundaries of all illnesses, even influencing the diagnoses provided by doctors.[10] The interpretations family members give to matters of cause, cure, and control are also at the core of their decision-making about how best to deal with the sick person in their lives. Although it constitutes the unofficial ideology of the McLean's Family and Friends support group, it is no easy thing for healthy family members truly to believe they had no part in causing a loved one's mental illness, can't cure it, and can't control it. Every person I interviewed for this book necessarily struggles with these issues. In Chapter 5, I look at how caregivers theorize about cause, cure, and control, and how their theories, in turn, profoundly affect their lives.

FIVE

The Four Cs

To hear them say that it's a brain disease, it's like, "Wow, that's great." It's like diabetes; just give them the medication and fix it. We went in [to the hospital] that day or the next . . . and he was put on medication. He was given Haldol, which is an antipsychotic. Okay, so here again I think, "Oh, medication—wonderful." You know, my husband was glad. I mean, "Oh, this is going to fix him. Everything will be fine."

SECRETARY, *age fifty-one, mother*

All human beings are theorists. We may not think of ourselves that way since we normally take our implicit theories largely for granted. Still, it would be impossible to live without practical theories about all sorts of things.[1] Parents, for example, cannot raise their children without some guiding principles about what constitutes humanness, how babies are made socially human, what they need in order to thrive, and certainly their own role in shaping their children's lives. Of course, there is no shortage of childrearing theories. People disagree about everything from the role of spanking in creating moral persons to the importance of reading stories aloud in order to develop a child's intelligence. Similarly, there are fundamental disagreements and competing theories about why people commit crimes and what to do about it, why people are on welfare and how governments ought to deal with them, just how men and women are different from each other and how that influences their relationships, and so on. Despite the inherent ambiguity that surrounds such issues, we must nevertheless raise our children, negotiate intimate relationships, decide whether we believe in capital punishment, and vote whether or not to rescind welfare benefits. We can only make collective and personal decisions about most things by theorizing.

As a social scientist, I'm obliged to treat my theorizing in a more self-conscious way than most people. It's my responsibility to piece together carefully collected data in order to generate a persuasive and compelling theory about one or another aspect of social life. Even while exercising every possible safeguard in collecting systematic data, social scientists must nevertheless live with the recognition that because of the sheer complexity of social life their theories are always tentative. They are for-the-time-being theories, theories to depend on until more persuasive ones come along. Despite the appearance otherwise in some social science discourse, we can never prove our theories. All we can do is gather data that allows us to embrace a theory as more or less plausible. In the face of uncertainty, confusion, and complexity all persons do the same thing as we social scientists. All of us proceed in life with multiple theories that direct our perceptions and actions. We simply cannot operate without these theories to guide us, however incomplete and tentative they may be.

This chapter is about the theories caregivers construct as they try to understand mental illness and formulate their own role in helping a loved one besieged by depression, manic-depression, or schizophrenia. Just as in other aspects of their lives, caregivers must construct theories to bring some order to family lives made chaotic by mental illness. In the face of great uncertainty and ambiguity, there are still multiple and daily decisions to make. Caregivers must decide how much faith to put in medical science. They must decide how to respond to an episode of psychosis or, less dramatically, to the more routinely troubling behaviors of an ill person. They have to decide how much emotional support to extend to a troubled person. As described in earlier chapters, they need to somehow draw boundaries of obligation. As long as they choose to remain connected to an emotionally ill person, caregivers must make ongoing daily decisions. To succeed they need to have some guiding ideas, beliefs, or theories about what mental illness is and what they can do about it.

It is not at all surprising that when the members of the Family and Friends group at McLean's hospital get together each week, the two hours somewhat resemble a university seminar on the meanings of mental illness. However, unlike a didactic seminar, every person in the room has his or her own stories to tell and lots of personal questions to ask. They come to the support group looking for viable theories about matters that especially confuse them. They also want to see how others will react to their own theories, many of them at a different stages of development and held with greater or lesser certainty. They are there as well to collect additional data by listening to others who already have had experiences they anticipate for themselves. They come together because they share a family problem that dominates their lives and often seems utterly intractable. Underneath all the talk, however, group members espouse an illness ideology[2] of sorts that provides them some guidance and comfort. As mentioned briefly in earlier chapters, it is virtually mandatory during each meeting for the group to mention the Four Cs. Like an indispensable ritual in a religious service, members recite in unison, "I didn't cause it. I can't cure it. I can't control it. All I can do is cope with it."

The Four Cs is an appealing set of ideas for group members because it articulates with three interconnected and widely shared cultural "vocabularies of motive" in the United States.[3] These vocabularies dominate Americans' thinking about themselves, their relationships, and broader events in the world. The Four Cs implicitly suggest theories of mental illness that combine elements of *science, therapy,* and *spirituality.* Together these themes constitute a compelling cultural brew that provides comfort and a measure of direction to people who cannot escape asking, "What is the essential nature of mental illness? How and why do people become mentally ill? Might I somehow have contributed to a family member's gross unhappiness? What is the right way to deal with a mentally ill person? What are the limits in my ability to help a family member in such awful pain? What do I need to do for myself in order to avoid being consumed by another person's extraordinary emotional distress?"

That they haven't caused another person's difficulty and can't cure it fits well with a biomedical, scientific view of the world. It fits with a disease model of mental illness. The disease or biochemical view of depression, manic-depression, or schizophrenia is far and away the dominant theory of these afflictions in psychiatric medicine and also among group members. Caregivers share a general consensus that their family members suffer from a brain disease. A frequently used analogy compares mental illness with diabetes. I often heard family members say, "You would certainly take insulin to deal with a hormonal imbalance and it only makes sense to take psychotropic drugs to deal with the chemical imbalances in the brain responsible for mental illness." Aside from providing a compelling simile, the disease notion has the happy effect of relieving both the ill person and caregiver from most, but not all, responsibility for having caused the problem.

The belief that ill persons must ultimately take control of their own problem fits with important elements of what Philip Rieff has called a "therapeutic culture."[4] In American society, popular writings by psychiatrists, psychologists, and advice columnists have taken on an influential role. Media appearances have made "mind-tinkers" such as Laura Schlesinger, Dr. Ruth Westheimer, and John Bradshaw instant celebrities. Their appeal attests to the pervasive anxiety about questions of identity and psychological well-being in the society. Such "experts" are constantly dispensing prescriptions for happiness, sexual fulfillment, or mental health.[5]

Part of the contemporary therapeutic ideology is the notion that individuals are responsible for "getting their own heads straight." More important still is the pervasive idea that too deep an involvement with emotionally ill people generates a distinctive "disease" of its own—co-dependency. In *Codependent No More*, a book that has sold more than three million copies, Melody Beattie promises important, possibly lifesaving advice.[6] Her book's subtitle offers to tell persons ill with co-dependency *How to Stop Controlling Others and Start Caring for Yourself.* Along these lines, a family member's mental illness raises very fundamental questions for caregivers about how to help a loved one without "enabling" his or her illness.

The more I have thought about the Four Cs the more I see them as also having a kind of spiritual, Buddhist-like cast. Buddhists advocate that we stop trying to control everything in our lives, that we accept suffering as an integral part of life, and that we embrace our interconnectedness with all of nature. The Four Cs could easily have been written by the theologian and philosopher Thomas Moore who, in his book *Care of the Soul,* writes that "a major difference between care and cure is that cure implies the end of trouble . . . but care has a sense of ongoing attention. There is no end. Conflicts may never be fully resolved. . . . Awareness can change, of course, but problems persist and never go away. . . . Care of the soul . . . appreciates the mystery of human suffering and does not offer the illusion of a problem-free life."[7] However, despite nearly full agreement that their caregiving should be bounded by the truth of the Four Cs, group discussion always revealed how difficult it is for caregivers to really believe that they are not implicated in the cause of a loved one's illness, cannot be part of a cure through their actions, or cannot exercise any control over the person and the illness. They all, however, agree easily with the one affirmative piece of the mantra: they desperately need to find ways to cope with the rigors of caring for someone they love with mental illness.

The Four Cs point to the most essential problems of theory construction when it comes to caring for any ill person, but especially someone with mental illness. Dealing with mental illness is an ongoing exercise in navigating ambiguity because, despite medicine's claims to knowledge, no one really has a satisfactory way to think about cause and cure. If medicine did have an absolute handle on cause and cure, there would be no need for support groups and Four C-type dictums. Despite the best efforts of doctors, mental illness is still a mystery and how best to deal with it remains elusive. Unlike most physical illnesses, mental illnesses have a cloudy status. Critiques of the diagnostic categories used by psychiatrists reveal the socially constructed nature of mental illnesses.[8] Diagnosis is often difficult because therapists of all sorts do not agree on where the boundaries of normal behavior leave off and disease begins. Sufferers often get as many labels as the number of therapeutic experts they consult.

Because the next chapter, "Surviving the System," focuses on the difficulties caregivers have in managing various mental health bureaucracies and the people who inhabit them—a problem in coping really—I will hold off discussion of the fourth C until then. To further our immediate discussion, readers need to recognize that questions of cause, cure, and control are hard to untangle. Theories about cause bleed into beliefs about cure. In turn, ideas about what causes mental illness and whether a cure might be forthcoming deeply influence caregivers' judgments about the possibility of controlling the illness. Although I will try to catch the way cause, cure, and control intersect, orderly presentation requires that I separate them for purposes of analysis. The remainder of this chapter describes the way that people I interviewed grope toward workable theories of the causes of mental illness, the likelihood of ever curing it, and their appropriate role in trying to control it.

Cause

If there is a dominant or master narrative to the way caregivers think about the cause of mental illness, it is a biological view that understands mental illness as arising from chemical imbalances in the brain. It is not surprising that biology constitutes the dominant paradigm of explanation since the language of genetics and biological determinism currently frames discussion in the United States about all kinds of behaviors.[9] The contemporary primacy of genetic explanation represents a renaissance in biological thinking. The nineteenth century was "Darwin's century" since his theory of evolution so thoroughly shaped ideas about both physical and human nature.[10] During the early 1900s, however, the insights of cultural anthropology challenged the view that nature determines all. Rather than biology being our destiny, the new view was that culture is destiny.[11] Such a view prevailed for several decades, while coexisting uneasily with the apparent reality that we are, after all, living, breathing, biological animals.

The so-called nature/nurture debate has taken yet another turn in the last couple of decades. Biological thinking has made a big comeback as scientists have achieved extraordinary progress in understanding human genetics. Newspaper headlines trumpet the successes of scientists in cloning sheep and now serious debates ensue about the real possibility of duplicating human beings. Advances in genetics are making it possible for people to choose the sex of their children. With the advent of computer technologies, scientists appear to have the tools necessary for mapping all human genes. Related to these discoveries are advances in knowledge about a range of genetically determined diseases. We regularly hear that scientists are on the cusp of discovering the genes responsible for problems like sickle-cell anemia, various cancers, and developmental disabilities. We seem on the brink of a brave new world where biological explanations will be found for the full panoply of human ills. It is in the context of these scientific and public conversations that claims to the biological basis for mental illness are heard.

Every now and then there is news that scientists are close to finding the gene responsible for manic-depression or that fundamental discoveries in brain research will unlock the secrets of schizophrenia.[12] Psychiatry has evolved from a discipline seeking cures in talk into a science dedicated to chemical intervention, just as in every other branch of medicine. Now, there are psychopharmacologists whose expertise lies solely in the diagnoses of mental illnesses and the prescription of the "right" medications. No more talk, just the determination of the appropriate chemicals for particular symptoms. Even though the claims to scientific progress are not matched by definitive discoveries of the biochemical basis for mental illness,

patients and family members, like most Americans, have faith in
the medical rhetoric that it is only a matter of time before we learn
the organic causes of mental illness. Given these cultural and scientific developments, it is sensible that the language of biological
disorder would be the central pillar of caregivers' theories of
causation.

> Yeah, I definitely think it's . . . like wires are crossed. Her perception
> is just so off that I really believe that it's a body chemistry thing.
>
> ACCOUNTANT, *age thirty-five, daughter*

↩

> As I got to read more and more literature on genetic research on
> schizophrenia I found out that schizophrenia certainly has huge ge-
> netic components. . . . There is no question that I look at all mental
> illness as rooted in some chemical imbalance, except for some mild
> anxiety or situational depression, or something that is very concrete.
> But, for the most part, I think it's a biological component. For ex-
> ample, in my case, my brother and I who were raised in the same
> household were exposed to pretty much the same elements at a cer-
> tain time together. Yet, why is it that one is very different from the
> other? So, I strongly believe that it's genetic.
>
> SOCIAL WORKER, *age thirty-seven, son*

↩

> From what I gather from the literature it's . . . a chemical imbalance.
> It's nothing that the person did or didn't do. It's no fault of their
> own. They're just unfortunate to get it.
>
> TELEPHONE COMPANY EMPLOYEE, *age forty-two, husband*

Often, conversation about biological causation is coupled with
accounts of family genealogy. Once a family member becomes ill
and is diagnosed, caregivers typically embark on an archeological
excavation of family madness. Nearly always, "discoveries" of other
disturbed persons in their extended families follows on the diag-

nosis of their spouse, child, parent, or sibling. Questions are asked and histories sought. Through this process the pieces of a puzzle seem to come together, at least partly. After all, there was cousin Joe or aunt Pheobe or grandma Sara who was depressed, hospitalized for a "nervous breakdown," or was alcoholic, "probably to self-medicate for the pain of mental illness." In most interviews respondents reviewed family history from the perspective of biological pathology, as was the case of a real estate agent who said: "Let me tell you a little about his father . . . because of the genetic thing. On his father's side they all drank heavily—the father, the mother, the brother. I know my father drank, but none of us were alcoholics or whatever. But on George's side they were alcoholics. They were also a little off-the-wall totally."

I have no interest in trying to reject biological theories of mental illness. In fact, many of the genealogies described by respondents were enormously persuasive. Theirs were families in which several people had been diagnosed and treated for mental illness. In several instances, respondents were dealing with multiple family members struck down by depression, bipolar illness, or schizophrenia—one or more ill children, an ill spouse and children, a sibling and a parent, a child as well as a parent, and so on. It may very well be that purely biological theories will one day triumph over mental illness in quite the same way that the Salk vaccine eradicated polio. I certainly hope for this. At the same time, we need to view the "data" provided on family histories with some caution. Once people have a theory to guide them, they will most surely find evidence to fit that theory.

As we evaluate the theoretical perspectives of professionals, patients, and caregivers, we need to consider the "law of the hammer." If you give a child a hammer, he or she will no doubt find nails to bang. We simply need to consider that the prevailing view of mental illness as a brain disease predisposes caregivers to find data supporting that theory. People are prone to search out data supporting one or another of their theories while dismissing data that do not. Having offered this caveat, it should be said the people interviewed for this study nearly always advocated a multicausal model of mental illness. They typically began by expressing the importance of faulty brain chemistry, but, after some prodding, articulated a view that included elements of both nature and nurture.

> If you see something [passed] down in a family and it seems to be somehow a component in that family, a trait that is passed down, you always wonder like, "Oh, is it the family structure itself and how they interact and how it's set up that is really just perpetuating it or is there something biological happening?" I definitely believe that there is some sort of biological component that could be passed down, but I think, as well, that there definitely has to be something going on in the environment to trigger certain things.
>
> GRADUATE STUDENT, *age twenty-eight, wife*

↪

> I do believe it is a brain disease. But, you know, now I wonder. . . . My son went to China and used drugs there. Well, he also used drugs in college. In China, he said he used Turkish hashish, and he was drunk a lot. I mean, all of that I'm sure played a part somehow in this. I told you that he was constantly, from like fourth grade on, he was made fun of, and he was teased. And I think that probably influenced him. I think, you know, you've got both [nature and nurture].
>
> SECRETARY, *age fifty-one, mother*

↪

> I believe that depression is a chemical thing. I just read an article that the brain looks different for people who are depressed. I know it has a lot to do with serotonin levels and all of that, but I also think that sometimes there can also be things in somebody's past that trigger it or brings it out. I do think that's the case for David. My older brother actually molested him. And, I think that had a lot to do with it.
>
> ASSISTANT PRINCIPAL, *age forty-five, sister*

〜

Obviously he has the gene [for manic-depression], but then if something traumatic happens to you it's going to set it off.

ADMINISTRATIVE SECRETARY, *age fifty-three, mother*

As my conversation with each person moved along, the number
of possible causes mentioned for mental illness expanded. Along
with general agreement that family members have a genetic pre-
disposition or vulnerability to depression, manic-depression, or
schizophrenia, family members named a range of environmental
factors that presumably activated, triggered, or set off the bad biology. Their theorizing often employed the logic of proximate cause.
So, if a spouse lost a job some months prior to the onset of illness,
that was claimed, often with great certainty, as the environmental
trigger in the nature/nurture equation. Or, if a parent discovered
that a child had been experimenting with street drugs prior to an
episode of psychosis, this was seized upon as having precipitated
the event. Often, respondents were unshakable in their belief about
causation. Once caregivers settled on a particular environmental
variable as the culprit, they became hypervigilant about its presence.
The parent who believes street drugs to be responsible for a child's
problems greatly expands efforts to monitor his or her possible drug
use.

My point is that human beings often construct their theories on
exceedingly particularistic grounds. They see something that looks
like an important proximate cause and that becomes an essential
link in their causal model. As a matter of fact, such particularistic
versions of mental illness's cause often create problems in their
encounters with other family members and therapeutic experts. On
several occasions respondents expressed distress when their "theory" was rejected by the ill person, by other family members, or
by doctors. These caregivers believed that their closeness to the situation of the ill person—their intimacy with the data, I might say
—warranted that their theory be privileged over others. They

honestly felt that they were privy to events that gave them greater
insights into cause than was possible for more distant observers.
Just as scientists debate, even fight over, their theories at professional meetings, family members were often at odds about interpretations of cause and, thereby, about how to manage the problem. Here is an account of family conflict generated by competing
theories:

> This is hard because in the last [family therapy] meeting my sister
> said, "Well I see myself as the person who never did anything to get
> attention when I was a kid and I never asked for anything and I am
> afraid to ask for anything because I won't get it." ... And so I just
> said, "That is a flawed perception that is preventing you from mov-
> ing on and living your life." I said, "You see your childhood that
> way" and I said, "What I remember of our childhood, I just don't
> see it that way. Your way of seeing may be your way of seeing it,
> but it's preventing you from seeing who you are today and who you
> can be today and you are just not seeing it the way it was." And, of
> course, she got furious. "Who are you to judge me and say that what
> I am thinking is just a perception and what I think is what I think."
> And then my brother chimed up and said, "I agree with Michelle."
> And that is essentially what started it [family conflict].
>
> TECHNOLOGY LICENSER, *age thirty-three, sister*

Anger generated by competing theories was also occasionally evident in the relationships between caregivers and therapists of various sorts. Finding Dr. Right is no easy task for both emotionally
ill patients and their caregivers. Because the causes of mental illness
are cloudy, therapists can be judged as "bad" if they seem to have
"off-the-wall" theories. Patients will often dump therapists who
seem to be emphasizing things that they judge as off the point. In
several cases, spouses and parents were upset that a husband, wife,
or child was listening to a therapist's version of cause that they
thought was just plain wrong. At least when it comes to talk therapy, a criterion for judging quackery is the therapist's commitment

to a theory discrepant from one's own. As an example, one wife was extremely upset that she and her husband were paying lots of money to a therapist who wanted to explore the untimely death of her husband's dad:

> Ted has had a lot of help with psychiatrists and psychologists. Some of them who were just no good. One guy was completely convinced Ted was depressed because he lost his father when he was seven years old. [I know that] Ted was depressed because he had lost his job and his lifestyle at the age of 32. . . . So anyway . . . Ted was continuing to see this gentleman. A half hour is nothing. Because you just get into something and "whoops, time to go." And this was like, "Time to go, see you." And . . . all he wanted to do [was] psychoanalysis on Ted. He wanted to talk about the family and the father that died when Ted was seven. That's not what Ted needed. Ted's depression didn't stem back from a childhood trauma. It stemmed from an illness two years earlier.
>
> CUSTOMER REPRESENTATIVE, *age thirty-five, wife*

The widespread availability of a biomedical, disease, or broken brain rhetoric to explain mental illness *generally* has the effect of insulating caregivers from feelings of blame. If caregivers believe that an ill family member is essentially plagued by bad biology, such a view *largely* protects them from feeling somehow personally blameworthy. However, among those who held most steadfastly to biological explanations were parents who, although healthy themselves, felt guilty for having passed along the offending mental illness genes to their sick children. The possibility, if not the likelihood, of genetic inheritability also created problems for healthy children who had to decide what to tell prospective partners ("Who's really going to want to marry into the genes I have?") and for parents who worry about becoming grandparents ("I always used to think . . . I'd love to be a grandparent, but now I'm thinking I'm not sure I want to have grandchildren."). One woman found it distressing to contemplate the genetic transmission of mental illness because she worried about her own health. Even more, though, she worried about her young child's future ("I don't want to think about it . . . I know my whole life I will be worried about his mental health . . . Maybe mental illness is just around the corner.").

Pure disease versions of cause limit caregiver blame to the oblique possibility that they passed along faulty genes. However, once environmental factors enter into the calculus of cause, the door for blaming caregivers is thrown wide open. Having acknowledged that mental illness might be related to stress, to life disappointment, to an accretion of social injuries, to such traumas as divorce, or to a range of developmental problems in childhood, caregivers are inevitably led to assess their culpability. Parents, mothers in particular, are especially likely to ruminate about the possibility that the misery of mental illness might be traced to their personal failures.

As I write these words, a book entitled *The Nurture Assumption*, claiming that parenting has little significance in determining the fate of children, has kicked off a voluble enough debate to have reached the public media.[13] My own view is that the conversation will be short-lived, both because there are too many flaws in the book's argument and because it is so deeply ingrained a cultural assumption in the United States that, for better or worse, parents significantly mold their children. Although another book no longer has nearly the hold on American parents that it once did, the ideas in Dr. Benjamin Spock's *The Common Sense Book of Baby and Child Care* first published in 1946, remain influential.[14] Spock proposed that mothers were literally responsible for shaping their children's personalities. "Deep in their hearts most middle-class, Spock-taught mothers believed that if they did their job well enough, all their children would be creative, intelligent, kind, generous, happy, brave, spontaneous, and good—each, of course, in his or her own special way."[15] While mothers might now reject the rigidly deterministic version of Spock's views, they must nevertheless contemplate their possible role in causing a child's illness.

Well, [about] cause. I mean, sometimes [I feel] I may have caused it. I may have, but it's not something that kills me with guilt. . . . I think I was a good parent to him. . . . I mean, I know he is having issues because I mother-smother, but it's only because . . . he needs that . . . He needs someone to mother him.

ADMINISTRATIVE SECRETARY, *age fifty-three, mother*

⌇

One of the hardest things for me before she was diagnosed was not knowing what I was doing wrong as a mother. You know, she had been through a couple of my depressions. She had been through [my] hard divorce. I mean, she has a grandmother who is schizophrenic, but, come on, she was a really nice kid until she was fifteen and ran away. Why is she so horrible now? How come I don't know this kid anymore? I mean why is she hanging out with troublemakers and why is she not coming home at night and why is she lying to me all the time? This is not the kid that I raised. Was I the problem? When she was diagnosed I could finally separate her mental illness from my parenting, but it took years of soul searching to reach that level of understanding.

GRADE SCHOOL TEACHER, *age forty-eight, mother/daughter*

⌇

I hoped for all my children, for them just to be happy, because as a child . . . I was afraid a lot. I was unhappy a lot. And I just did not want that for my children. I thought, "This (parenting) is something I can do right. I can have happy children. I can provide an atmosphere for them where they will just be happy and healthy." And now we have a terrible illness. . . . I blame myself for not recognizing it sooner. I think I should have been more aware of it [his problem]. I was wrong.

SECRETARY, *age fifty-one, mother*

Feelings of blame or guilt, like every emotion, can arise only in social context. Self-feelings are intimately connected to the way we believe others are evaluating us. Charles Horton Cooley, a turn-of-the-century sociologist, coined the term the "looking-glass self" to convey the idea that others serve as mirrors in which we see ourselves reflected.[16] There is no way to experience such reactions as shame or guilt without introspectively evaluating and appraising our own behavior while taking into account the actions of others. It is in this sense that our "self" is both the subject and the object of our own acts. We engage in a behavior as an acting subject. We then introspectively evaluate the meaning of that behavior to ourselves and to others based on the responses they have made to it. Such internal evaluations then influence our future course of action. The ability of persons to both act and reflect on their actions from various perspectives lies at the root of what is distinctively human.

Whether or not we agree with them, the evaluations of others affect us deeply. Caregivers, while angered by the unreasonable judgments of others, could not easily slough off their evaluations. They discovered that they had to live with a whole chorus of onlookers who were playing the blame game. During a recent meeting of the Family and Friends group there was an animated discussion about "outsiders" who heaped blame from a distance. Family members felt profoundly misunderstood by people who knew little about the day-to-day realities of caring for a mentally ill person, but still held them responsible for the upsetting behaviors of their ill spouse, child, sibling, or parent. After years of defending themselves against unsolicited and negative opinions, some caregivers adapted by significantly restricting their contact with well-meaning but ignorant family members or friends. One woman said that she now divides the world into those who "get it" and those who don't. She will only discuss her caregiving plight with people who know about mental illness firsthand or who can listen without making moral judgments.

However much they restrict their interactions, caregivers cannot fully insulate themselves from charges of irresponsibility. They have to contend with the fact that observers, although distant from the nitty-gritty details of their lives, still construct their own theories of mental illness and caregiving. They might be theories hastily and thoughtlessly constructed, built from incomplete data, or created from thoroughly misguided stereotypes of mental illness. Still, they are theories that frame their responses to caregivers and, therefore, inevitably influence how caregivers see themselves. At every turn, caregivers find themselves judged. The judgments can come from the sick person in their care:

[My husband kept saying], "There's nothing wrong with me, it's you. If you weren't the way you are, I wouldn't be the way I am." So for years I thought it was me. . . . That's how I felt and I never told anyone . . . outside our immediate family. I never discussed it with anyone. Once in a while I'd talk to his mother and I would get a remark like, "You must be doing something wrong." So, it's me. It had to be me. You think, "If I don't do this, then maybe he won't yell." So I won't do it. "If I don't say this, then he won't yell." . . . Eventually, you stop talking and you go within yourself and then you know what happens? You shut down and that is what I did. I shut down.

DAY-CARE ATTENDANT, *age fifty-five, wife*

The judgments can come from uncomprehending members of an extended family who don't really understand the circumstances facing caregivers:

My mother-in-law and father-in-law, Anita's parents, are coming up for Thanksgiving. It's gonna be very interesting because they think it's [daughter's illness] a fabrication. The way my father-in-law sees it, she needs to get her ass kicked royally. He's into severe punishment. My mother-in-law isn't any better.

ART RESTORER, *age fifty, father*

The judgments can come from public officials, like police, who become involved in managing a bad episode:

Like we had an episode where the police showed up at the house, and they're like, "Look, do something." I'm like, "Hey, what do you

want me to do? There is nothing that I can do." I'm really upset at
the ignorance of these people that make it so much more difficult
for her, for me, for everybody involved. Basically, you know, he was
this young cop and . . . he was just very [demanding]. You know,
"Do something!" He said, "This house [she's living in] should be
condemned." I'm like, "Great!" Here I am thinking, "I want her out
of here as much as anybody else and I can't get her out." She doesn't
want to stay there but she doesn't want to go anywhere else and I
can't get her anywhere. What am I going to do, pay for an apartment
for her? I can't. And if she went there, she'd be so delusional they'd
probably throw her out. So I feel like she's living in this place that
I don't even like to be because it's just so dilapidated. It's too depressing for me to just sit there. And she lives that life and it's just
so hard and that's one of the big things that I have been trying to
deal with. And here he [policeman] is trying to give me a hard time.
[*imitating the policeman*] "You see this house and you don't do
something? Can't you get her some help?" They [police] didn't want
to come back. They were going to put her in protective custody. . . .
Some therapist joked later with me, "What did they think, they'd
put her in protective custody, lock her up for the night and she'd be
cured in the morning?" It's ridiculous.

ACCOUNTANT, age thirty-five, daughter

Finally, the judgments can come from the therapeutic professionals who treat their ill family members:

He [psychiatrist] says, "There is this thing called 'expressed emotion.' " Here I am sobbing my heart out, right? She [daughter] is
going into the hospital and she is not safe and he says, "And you
need to stop doing expressed emotion or you are going to alienate
this kid." And I looked at him and I said, "Don't you go there!" I
said, "Don't you dare blame this victim because I won't have it!"
How dare he watch me sob my heart out about this kid that isn't
safe and say, "You need to stop doing expressed emotions."

PHYSICAL THERAPIST, age forty-nine, mother

I have already mentioned several times that feelings of responsibility and obligation are not equally distributed in American society. Women, far more than men, are seen as primarily responsible for caring when a family member becomes ill. Caring is so thoroughly constructed as women's work that "women are themselves drawn into participation in prevailing relations of inequality."[17] Rather than questioning their own far greater involvement in all aspects of caregiving, women have internalized cultural definitions that define caring as central to women's role within the family. By "doing the work of 'wife' and 'mother,' women quite literally produce family life from day to day, through their joint activities with others. By 'doing family' in traditional ways, houshold members sustain and reproduce the 'naturalness' of prevailing arrangements."[18]

As you have seen, the women I interviewed often described feeling guilty for not caring "enough" and then find that blame for "inadequate" care is nearly always directed at them. None of the men I interviewed expressed guilt about not caring enough and seldom were they burdened by other people's accusations that they were doing a poor caregiving job. The sociologist Antonio Gramsci offered the term "cultural hegemony" to refer to the variety of social processes through which persons are trained to give assent to the social arrangements that oppress them.[19] The term certainly applies well to the caregiving circumstances of women. Women do more caregiving than men. They themselves believe that they ought to care more. They feel guilty when they can't meet impossible standards. Then, they are often blamed by onlookers when a mentally ill person becomes too troublesome. It is a destructive cultural feedback loop that sustains gender inequality and deepens the pain of dealing with an already impossible situation.

Anyone who takes a basic course in sociology or psychology learns about the nature/nurture debate. For most people the debate remains at an abstract level, removed from the stuff of daily life. However, for those suffering from mental illness and their families, efforts to learn whether mental illness is explained by biology or environment are not dispassionate intellectual exercises. In the end, for reasons I have explained, nearly everyone with whom I spoke favored biochemically based theories to explain depression, manic-depression, or schizophrenia. However, like social scientists who need to think long and hard about the issue, caregivers also understand that while all illness symptoms are "biochemically mediated, that does not make [them] biochemically caused."[20] Nearly all feel obliged to modify exclusively biomedical theories with some version of the view that mental illness arises from an elusive concatenation of biology, temperament, life events, and social environment. The adoption of more complex theories made caregivers more vulnerable to blame for a family member's problem. It also diminished their hopes that a cure for mental illness might be forthcoming any time soon.

Cure

Patty is a physical therapist who speaks frequently in this book. I met her at the Family and Friends group and since our interview about a year ago we've maintained casual contact. Just recently, she called to invite me to a gala celebration of her fiftieth birthday and Johanna's high school graduation. At the time of our interview she never thought Johanna would finish high school and even feared that her daughter might die from her illness. The party was a wonderful event, attended, it turned out, by some other people interviewed for this book, among them a grade school teacher named Grace who had another success story for me. In fact, Grace asked if we might once again talk since her perspective had so thoroughly changed in a year's time. It seems that her daughter, Alice, has also made a significant turnabout. Both daughters have stopped denying their illness, now faithfully comply with medication, and are holding down jobs they enjoy. Grace felt that it was important to amend her earlier story that left off with a sense of exhaustion and fatalism about the likelihood of Alice's ever emerging from the encompassing shadow of mental illness.

The good news from both mothers was, of course, heartening.

Their updates also reminded me that my interviews only catch people at a particular moment in time. It could be that the individuals most motivated to participate in this study are those most thoroughly caught up in the turbulence of a family member's mental illness. Patty's and Grace's continuing narratives suggest the possibility that mental illness stories can end happily. Naturally, I hope that their daughters continue to thrive, but the range of accounts I've now heard, in writing both *Speaking of Sadness* and this book, cause me worry on their behalf. One of the insidious features of mental illness is its pattern of periodic retreat and eventual return, sometimes with greater ferocity. Like a mutating virus that lies dormant somewhere deep in our bodies, the illness generates cycles of hope and disappointment by causing sufferers and those who love them to mistake remission for cure. In her recent book, *Prozac Diary*, Lauren Slater describes in beautiful prose the shattering disappointment of her illness's return after a year's respite.[21] Following a lifetime of depression and obsessive-compulsive behavior, punctuated by five hospitalizations, Prozac had miraculously "cured" her. The cure, however, ended abruptly on a trip to Kentucky for work on her Master's thesis:

> First I had a mini-anxiety attack . . . and then I started having trouble sleeping, and then, one morning, two weeks into my Kentucky trip, I woke up a madwoman again. The Prozac had simply stopped working. That's impossible. No, it's not. I started to tap and touch things and to have to count until my mind clenched closed. Where are you, Prozac? Come home, come home. Back to my body again. This, I now know, is what boozers must feel when they drop a full bottle and it breaks against the ground. Or what women must feel when their husbands leave for bagels on a Sunday morning and later drop a line from Katmandu. When you fall so deeply in love, when you have, with great consideration, tied the slow satin knot, you don't expect to be betrayed. But then you are. . . . Crack-ups are always terrible, but this one was so sudden, so complete. . . . My mental illness came rushing back in. As fast as Prozac had once, like

a sexy firefighter, doused the flames of pain, the flames now flared back up, angrier than ever, and my potent pill could do nothing to quell the conflagration.[22]

The conversations I had with family members about cure reflected the yin-yang of human beings' response to desperate situations. Caregivers tried to balance reason about the likely permanence of mental illness with hope for a cure. That is, their images of the future, their own and their loved one's, were a product of both head and heart. Their theories about cure were tied to the length of a family member's history with mental illness and the number of times high hopes had already been dashed. At the beginning of things, when mental illness is a relative stranger, caregivers have great optimism that medical science can beat back the monster. Along the way, those hopes are pushed aside by a resigned belief that mental illness might very well never leave home. Even at its worst, though, family members typically hold onto remnants of hope that somehow medical science will find a way to save themselves and their ill children, spouses, parents, or siblings. The combination of head and heart, reason and emotion, shapes their subjective experiences and, thus, their theories about cure. Here are typical expressions of hope caregivers felt on the occasion of mental illness's debut appearance:

We had a magic wand. The pills are going to make everything fine. Even though people told me that the pills were not magic. The intellectual and the emotional realities were not totally connected yet.
GRADE SCHOOL TEACHER, *age forty-eight, mother/daughter*

⌒

I definitely wanted him [brother] to get better. I kind of had this feeling that it was just gonna stop. I had this belief that finally he was gonna go somewhere and get help. I was like, "That's it. If he gets help, things will be okay. . . . Yeah." I just thought that it would be over with. It wasn't something that I'd have to deal with the year after or the next year. Because I really didn't have any clue of what to call this, you know what I mean? He had no idea what bipolar was or anything like that. None of us really did. My mom's a really quiet person. She told us about it, but . . . she'd just say things that would make us feel better. So, she was saying things like he was gonna get better, "He'll get help, and he'll be fine." And my dad was kind of the same way too. But, he knew that something had gone wrong. It's just not gonna go away like my mom was thinking, you know?

STUDENT, *age nineteen, sister*

↩

Of course, as a mother of someone who is schizo-affective, which is schizophrenia plus an affective disorder, to hear them say that it's a brain disease, it's like, "Wow, that's great." It's like diabetes; just give them the medication and fix it. We went in [to the hospital] that day or the next, I think it was the next morning, and he was put on medication. He was given Haldol, which is an antipsychotic. Okay, so here again I think, "Oh, medication—wonderful." You know, my husband was glad. I mean, "Oh, this is going to fix him. Everything will be fine."

SECRETARY, *age fifty-one, mother*

↩

The first time it happened we thought maybe this is just a fluky thing, a once in a lifetime thing.

RETIRED SECRETARY, *age fifty-eight, mother*

In my research methods classes, I try to teach students about the logic of "analytic induction."[23] I tell them that field-workers, like anthropologists immersed in a foreign culture, must begin to construct tentative theories as soon as they enter their new worlds. At first, flooded by events, situations, and behaviors that they have never seen before, their theories will inevitably be highly tentative and fairly simple. Still, researchers must do their best to make sense of things, to offer some initial explanations for what they are seeing. As time passes and their new culture becomes more familiar, they will reject completely some of their initial ideas, decide that other lines of thinking have promise and should be elaborated, and begin to construct yet additional theories. In this way, analytic induction involves a process of ongoing theory refinement until researchers create explanations that, ideally, are no longer contradicted by new data. Although caregivers have been involuntarily and abruptly dropped into a new and baleful culture, their effort to make sense of things still approximates the logic of fieldwork. Like anthropologists, they begin their caregiving as strangers in a strange land.

Part of family members' initial confusion is the difficulty of getting precise information (data) about what is going on. Their situation approximates that of the anthropologist who does not really speak the new culture's language and has a tough time getting the natives to cooperate in explaining even the simplest rituals. Caregivers often had trouble comprehending the resistance of professionals who seemed unwilling to give even the barest information required to make sense of things. "The doctors," one father explained, "didn't want to talk to us. Well, here is this young kid and he's over twenty-one and who are we? Nobody really wanted to talk to us. We needed information. We wanted to know what was going on and nobody would tell us." A young woman had a similar problem, saying, "We didn't really understand it. We're in shock. We didn't have that much support as far as information." And a mother complained, "You know, I don't know much about the mental health field, but [what they said] seemed silly to me. When he was discharged they said to us, 'Oh, he had a breakdown.' I thought, 'a breakdown'??"

It doesn't take long for family members to reject their first, wildly optimistic theory of a quick fix for the problem that forced them into an alien world of psychiatry, social workers, psychotropic drugs, and locked wards. When they did finally get doctors to explain things, messages of hope were tempered by the communication that a regimen of medication and therapy would only make their child, spouse, parent, or sibling "functional." Rarely did doctors speak the language of absolute cure. A husband trying to comprehend what to expect after his wife's first psychotic episode said, "Early on, her doctor told me, 'Here's the deal, we can figure out what's causing it and stabilize it.' I actually appreciated the doctor's frankness." Such communications required a conceptual shift in caregivers' consciousness as they now had to understand mental illness as a chronic, long-term problem. Such a dour change in thinking was hard to adopt until they experienced one or more cycles of hope and disappointment.

> We kept hoping that she'll pass through it and you know, maybe that's wishful thinking. She goes back and forth, back and forth and you get high hopes. You go along for three or four weeks and then all of a sudden it starts over again and I don't see any light ahead at all. They put her on [names drug] and she was on it for three and a half months and she was doing beautifully until a month ago.
>
> HOMEMAKER, *age seventy-two, mother*

↩

> By that point it was probably like just two years of her . . . being really bad. We were all just kind of like waiting for her to . . . snap out of it or [we were] just kind of thinking that things were starting to get better somehow. I mean, it's very easy to make yourself think that things are turning around.
>
> RESEARCH ASSISTANT, *age twenty-three, daughter*

↩

> I actually think that the first six or eight months of her [being] on medication were very good months and I felt like it was going to be fine forever and then when it fell apart the first time it was ten times worse than any other falling apart before.
>
> GRADE SCHOOL TEACHER, *age forty-eight, mother*

Occasionally, social scientists are seduced by their own theories. They become so emotionally attached to their ideas, so in love with them, that the prospect of changing theories or leaving them behind is hard to contemplate. As one wag put it, "Even a brutal gang of facts is sometimes not enough to murder a cherished theory." Texts on doing research typically have substantial discussions about the problems researchers sometimes have maintaining their objectivity. When participant observers lose their analytical detachment and too thoroughly identify with the cultures they are trying to understand, they are said to have "gone native." Caregivers share much in common with researchers who have gone native, lost the ability for dispassionate detachment, and no longer strive for objectivity. Because of the love that binds kin, caregivers are emotionally unable to abandon hope for a cure. Still, even as they express them, respondents realize that there is an air of unreality about their wishes for a cure.

> I'm always latching on to something that will save him. . . . I feel like I have to do that. But it's hard for me to imagine [a solution] if he doesn't get somewhat better. I think he will. I think there is a lot of hope. See, I'm saying that now but then there are times when I feel hopeless about the whole thing.
>
> SECRETARY, *age fifty-one, mother*

⤳

> I don't know if it will ever be without medication that she'll be okay. Maybe she'll always have to be on an antipsychotic drug, I don't know. I sometimes think that if the right person came into her life who was a stronger male and was [a] more disciplined type of person, she would have financial security. These outside influences, I think, sometimes trigger what's happening with her. I think that maybe she could be okay. Maybe she could be okay. So, there is that hope. I know that she's going to be okay, even if she's going to have to go to the hospital every now and then.
>
> RETIRED SECRETARY, *age fifty-eight, mother*

⤳

> I sometimes have this fantasy that I would go into the woods and pick out herbs and have a science lab in the basement and I would

make a miracle drug and get my old [husband] back. Because there is a person inside of there. I saw it [illness] as a shell. And [it's] just a matter of tearing away [the shell] and once you do, he is there. You know what I mean?

STUDENT, age twenty-five, wife

Julia, a young wife with a three-year-old son, who just spoke, offers an imagery that I heard throughout these interviews. It is of a loving, whole, and healthy person lost to mental illness. It occurs to me that the metaphor of a "missing person" is an apt one for thinking about respondents' gradually fading hopes for a cure. When I have heard family accounts of actual missing persons on TV, the alternation over time of hope and disappointment that they describe parallels transformations in the way family caregivers regard the possibility of a cure.

In those tragic situations when a person is first discovered missing, there are labor-intensive searches to find them quickly. Initial searches are done with tremendous anxiety, but with a strong hope that the nightmarish problem will be quickly resolved. When the full-press efforts of family and police fail to find the person, the official search is eventually called off. It then becomes largely family members who must keep looking for the lost person, a task that they continue for some time with energy and dedication. Daily life, however, eventually blunts the kind of energy that can go into search efforts and hopes of a happy ending begin to erode significantly. As years go by without a trace of the missing person, family members are forced to acknowledge that their loved one is unlikely ever to be found. Now, left only with the memory of the person lost, they try their best to get on with their lives. Although they never completely abandon hope that the lost person will somehow reappear, they know in their hearts that the chances are slight. As the following comments illustrate, those who have lived for years with an ill family member have largely abandoned hope that their missing person will return.

This was just this absolutely beautiful daughter one day who [became] an absolute vegetable the next day. . . . With physical illness, medication or an operation or something would cure it. With this, there is nothing to cure it. . . . Risperidone [is] the thirteenth drug she's been on and at this point she's getting very unhappy. She's gained forty pounds. You wouldn't recognize her. If you take her off this medication . . . she'll end up back in the locked unit.

HOMEMAKER, *age seventy-two, mother*

⌒

This mental illness in my family has just been going on for so long that people [who] think that there is going to be a quick fix and the person is going to come back to quote unquote normal [are wrong]. I think when you talk about grief and loss, [it is] because people who are that ill [may] return to some level of functioning and positive living, but they may not ever get back to the son and daughter you knew before they had manic-depression.

TECHNOLOGY LICENSER, *age thirty-three, sister*

Reading what I have thus far written in this section, I feel slightly awkward about my own lines of analysis. In contrast to my emphases here, so many recent books offer optimism, hope, and the steps necessary to deal successfully with mental illness. Demetri and Janice Papolos have written a much cited book called *Overcoming Depression*.[24] A new book by Richard O'Connor is entitled *Undoing Depression*.[25] A range of personal memoirs describe the authors' victories over depression, manic-depression, and schizophrenia.[26] Julie Johnson's earlier book, *Hidden Victims*, is a bible of sorts in the Family and Friends support group, offering, as it does "an eight-stages healing process for the families and friends of mental illness."[27] I need to keep reminding myself that mental illnesses come in multiple hues, tones, and degrees and that the people I have interviewed may be dealing with family members who are at the most severely ill end of the continuum. I hope my own theorizing is not skewed by the failure to sufficiently highlight stories like the ones I heard from Patty and Grace about their daughters, or by a few people like Francine who described her husband's healing process this way:

> The more he is figuring out about his childhood, the more stable he becomes. He would be a perfect case to study because he really is figuring it out. You can actually see the progress, month by month I would say, or six months by six months. And he loves learning about that stuff and he's read a lot. . . . I think he's gonna be okay. And that's not just a pipe dream; I see him really working. . . . He was diagnosed four years ago and there would be little manic episodes, [but] they're just further and further apart all the time as he figures his life out.
>
> NURSE, *age fifty, wife*

I have tried to capture in these pages the most central threads in my interviews. With some exceptions, the stories largely convey an evolving pessimism among caregivers about the prospects for cure. Do they expect medical treatment to produce a measure of stability and functionality for the ill person in their lives? Yes! But a cure? No!

Now, we turn to the "third C"—"I can't control it." While it may be heartbreaking to watch someone they love unravel completely, caregivers presumably have no control over the mental illness. Although a good spiritual guideline, you will see that family members anguish over just how much to intervene in the lives of their ill child, spouse, parent, or sibling. If they do not intervene enough, the consequences for both the sick person and themselves could be disastrous, even fatal. If they intervene too much in order to save an ill person from themselves, they become "enablers." The matter of control is yet another conundrum for caregivers.

Control

Throughout I have been trying to build on the observation made in the first chapter that once we listen to an ill person's narrative, once we bear witness to their pain, we simultaneously change the direction, often radically, of our own lives. Early in the interviewing process for this book I realized that my conversations with caregivers had a different tone from the ones I had done years previously with depressed people. In retrospect, I see that ill people are largely absorbed by their own pain. In contrast, caregivers' conversation, while centered on their sick family member, nearly always incorporated talk about the impact of illness on their whole family, on other relatives and friends, on their own jobs, and on their own health. As I listened to them, I often pictured them, along with their families, as reluctant passengers in a car, forced into a thoroughly unwelcome journey without a clear destination, and always worried that the driver's disturbingly erratic behavior might potentially destroy them all. When mentally ill people lose control of their lives, so do those who love them. It is an intolerable condition and, therefore, not surprising that a caregiving priority is to somehow reestablish control.

People require order. We try to minimize ambiguity, unpredictability, and disorder. The matter of order is, in fact, central to my discipline. One definition might be that sociology is the study of how human beings collectively "accomplish" the production of social order.[28] We might very well think of society as an invention to ensure order, predictability, and a comforting measure of certainty. Social order, moreover, cannot be produced and sustained without social control. Commitment to a society involves submitting to a "social contract," as it were.[29] The contract requires that we give up a significant measure of personal freedom and subordinate ourselves to the demands of society. Social order and social control are also intimately connected in our everyday lives. When order is threatened, we try to exercise greater control over the disordering events or people.

While all traumas create chaos, intermittent and unpredictable traumas are the most terrorizing. For example, those political regimes that use torture to elicit information or confessions know that victims will break down most quickly if they can't predict when they will next be subject to physical or emotional violence. Although all illnesses create social and psychological disorder, mental illnesses are especially tortuous because they appear unpredictably and take unpredictable forms. Mentally ill people are unable to abide by even the most fundamental requirements of the social contract and thereby gravely threaten the intelligibility of everyday life. Caregivers, in turn, are forced into a state of unremitting hypervigilance as they wait for yet another crisis. The problems of restoring order are multiplied when caregivers reach the unhappy conclusion that they have little control *over the person's illness.*

Were we controlling Jack? Yes and no. We were controlling the part that wasn't psychotic. The psychotic part, I don't know that we had any control over. I think that we were just lucky that there was enough that wasn't psychotic. We were able to control enough of the situation to get him through these gauntlets.

RETIRED SCHOOLTEACHER, *age sixty-two, father*

～

I mean, I accept the fact that I have no control over her. . . . The acceptance is not so much that she is mentally ill. The acceptance is that I have no control over her. I can't prevent her from being a jerk or from being out of control or from making bad decisions. I have no control over her. . . . It took me two years to get there. I worked hard to get there. . . . When Alice is manic, she doesn't have any control over herself either. She doesn't remember what happened when she gets really manic. She has no organized memory of what took place so that she can't even learn from her mistakes or correct them or understand why she's dealing with the consequences that she is.

GRADE SCHOOL TEACHER, *age forty-eight, mother*

In earlier discussions, I pointed out that as caregivers try to modulate their negative feelings toward an ill family member, they make a crucial distinction between the illness and the person. To maintain warm feelings toward the person, they express their animosity toward the illness that has captured them. Although they sometimes wonder whether they are being manipulated in the name of illness, they nevertheless largely hold to the theory that the illness controls the individual. In turn, most caregivers say with sincerity, "I can't control the illness." Such a recognition requires a redirection of energy. Instead of trying somehow to control the illness, they strive to create order by *controlling the environment*. If they cannot alter a mental illness's course, they will make sure that all the pieces are in place to minimize the effects of the next bout with depression, delusional thinking, or mania. Caregivers achieve an important sense of efficacy and order by adopting a managerial or advocacy role.

This is one of the things that I said, "I'm going to be an advocate here at least. . . . [I will] at least figure out what is going on, take control of the situation." You know . . . I work with a lot of lawyers and a lot of different companies, and the experience, I am realizing, has taught me a way to take control of the situation. I've gotten better at managing.

ACCOUNTANT, *age thirty-five, daughter*

〜

I can't do anything about this mental illness as far as the illness is concerned, [but] I can control her environment. I cannot control this illness that is in her brain and I can't get in there. If I could, I would go in and I would pull out whatever it is. [But] I can control what the doctors are doing.

HOMEMAKER, *age seventy-two, mother*

〜

When she's in the hospital, I am on the phone to the morning shift, the afternoon shift, and the night shift, talking to the staff. I'm talking to everyone, "How is Jeanne today? What did she have for dinner? Who did she talk to? What medications has she had tonight?

Do you need to know anything from me?" Everybody knows that I'm calling.

RETIRED SECRETARY, *age fifty-eight, mother*

↩

It's not really control [I have], it's advocacy. It's getting the best you can from what you've got. And it's making sure that people don't fuck up.

PHYSICAL THERAPIST, *age forty-nine, mother*

↩

She [sister] basically withdrew. She went to the joint counseling sessions. I mean, you didn't have to force her to go, but she sat there and said nothing. So, she basically took a very withdrawn approach to it [brother's illness]. . . . I reacted totally different. I took charge of the whole situation. And I forced people to make decisions when decisions had to be made. It was easier for me to be able to do that than to just sit and watch because I can't stand it if I can't control something. And I couldn't just sit and watch, so we talked about how the fact that, during the times that he has had occurrences that have required us to react and respond, she has withdrawn and I have jumped in and taken charge.

TECHNOLOGY LICENSER, *age thirty-three, sister*

While generally believing that mental illness controls a person they love, such a theory is held somewhat tentatively because caregivers have also seen their spouse, child, parent, or sibling "pull it together" when they must. One mother, observing that her son can sometimes move in and out of psychosis when the situation demands it, asked out loud, "How does the mind go from out of control to control like this?" A daughter who felt angry about her father's illness told me, "There are times when he's lucid and he's just being manipulative." Such modifications of the theory that says mentally ill people have no control over their illness also creates problems with the wisdom of assuming too active a managerial role.

Caregivers worry that by too thoroughly managing the lives of their ill family members, they remove incentives for them to gain independence and manage their own lives. They worry, in other words, that the price of greater order through active management may be to "enable" a family member's illness.

Virtually all human relationships raise questions about the dialectic of dependence and independence. Every parent, for instance, must negotiate a delicate balance of autonomy and reliance, of distance and closeness with their children.[30] American parents generally see it as a personal failure if their children cannot gain independence at a relatively early age. At the same time, children are, by definition, dependent. Parents, therefore, must chart a course that both maximizes independence while creating a safety net in the event that children falter in their efforts to meet each new developmental and social task. As with much social life, and consequently with much compelling sociological analysis, it is contradiction, irony, and paradox that often best capture the complexity of things. Most human beings are independent and dependent at the same time. Caregivers hope that ill family members can eventually "find their own way in the world and develop confidence that they are strong enough to survive outside the protective family circle."[31] They know, however, that if they do not protect an ill person enough, the result is likely to be chaos and disorder. If, on the other hand, they protect an ill person too much they might be contributing to his or her illness.

MDDA group members frequently discuss the twin ideas of codependence and enabling. The conversation reflects the genuine confusion family members face in trying to decide just how much to help. Understandably, participants most usually invoke the codependency notion when individuals describe their own declining health because they have become so enmeshed in another person's illness. In these cases, group members are likely to emphasize the "I can't control it" injunction and describe in detail the problems of caring too much. They might echo the words of Melody Beattie, one of the gurus of the co-dependency movement, who writes, "I saw people who had gotten so absorbed in other people's problems that they didn't have time to identify or solve their own. These were people who had cared so deeply, and often destructively, about other people that they had forgotten how to care about themselves."[32]

The emotional tension felt by all caregivers is the simultaneous urge to "save" a loved one in trouble and to withdraw so that sick persons can better appreciate the consequences of their damaging behaviors. How much to help, that is the question! And it is a question that stumps caregivers throughout the course of their involvement with a sick family member. Perhaps the most complicated interpretive problem for caregivers is to achieve the correct balance between necessary help, efforts to control, and fostering independence. Although it sometimes takes a long time to understand it fully, most family members eventually comprehend the central paradox of caregiving. It is that by trying too hard to control another person's illness they become controlled by it. Such a lesson is particularly hard to learn because head and heart oppose each other. Withholding certain kinds of care is agonizing because to do so, although appearing rationally correct, feels emotionally wrong. Over and again, I heard family members describe their inability to "do the right thing."

> He [the doctor] made this prescription for me—ninety days I had to go to ALANON meetings for enablers. I didn't even know what it was. I said "What are you talking about? My son doesn't drink." He said "You are a classic enabler." . . . [But] I don't know how to change and I don't want to change. I don't want to be somebody different. I can't be a hard-nose with this child. . . . So this is why, when people say, "Take a stand, you've got to be tough," it's like I don't know how to do it.
>
> REAL ESTATE BROKER, *age forty-five, mother*
>
> ↩

> I couldn't not be there for someone who needed me. I couldn't. His needs are very great and one of the reasons that it was very difficult to make the right decisions about his illness was because he was also

a child and a teenager and to try to keep two tracks going at once [is hard]. You're the mother and, you know, you want to let them grow, make mistakes, be angry, whatever you need to do to just be normal in your relationship with them. On the other hand, he is sick and you are trying to protect them and give them extra support.

RETIRED BOOK EDITOR, *age fifty-one, mother*

In a few cases, caregivers had reached the point where they felt obliged to take a "tough-love" stand. As in so many other caregiving moments, family members who finally refuse to yet again bail a sick person out of trouble may be criticized even by those who presumably ought best to understand. One woman recounted for me the reaction of fellow support group members after describing her decision to take a "hard line" with her daughter who left home at eighteen. As I heard in so many other interviews, Patty had to decide whether to provide Johanna with financial support. At the time, her unemployed daughter was living with a struggling group of rock musicians. Here is how she described her daughter's request for help, her decision to withhold it, and the response of fellow caregivers:

"You know, I realize that she is eighteen and I have to let her go and I have to let her be responsible for her own care. And Ellen [a group member] said, "Well, how can you do that? She's sick." And I said, "I have no choice. She's eighteen. I did this last hurrah. I tried to get her in hospital. I can't. I have to let her go. I have to grieve this and let her go." And Ellen said, "But you have to take care of her and give her money and stuff." And I said, "Let me tell you, I had coffee with her last week and she asked me for ten dollars for food" and the whole room fell silent and they said, "And what did you do?" And I said, "I said 'no.'" And the whole room gasped and . . . half the people said, "Oh my God, that's the right thing to do but I never could have done it." Half the room said that. And I said, "Well, it was like this knife in my gut when I did it. It was like the hardest thing I ever did." And the other half of the room, in-

cluding Ellen, said, "How can you do that? She still needs you." And
I said, "No."

PHYSICAL THERAPIST, *age forty-eight, mother*

Decisions about appropriate levels of support are hard enough
to make when the refusal to help can result in a sick person's going
hungry. Caregivers also know that if they don't jump in to help, an
ill person may end up wandering the streets in a psychotic state,
may make terrible financial and relationship decisions, and sometimes may even land in jail. As awful as it is to contemplate these
outcomes, there is yet a worse scenario. Mental illness is for too
many sufferers a terminal condition. It has been conservatively estimated that 30,000 Americans suffering from mental illness commit suicide each year. However, because of inaccurate reporting,
the number could be as much as three times higher. Overall, mental
illness is the ninth leading cause of death across all age groups.[33]

The ultimate terror for family caregivers is that someone they
love will commit suicide. A high proportion of the respondents for
this book reported that a sick spouse, child, parent, or sibling had
already made a serious suicide attempt and they believed the person
in their care might very well try again. When family members cannot bring themselves to take vacations or to draw hard and fast
boundaries in order to prevent enabling, they often explain their
behaviors the same way that Nancy did in Chapter 2 when she said,
"I would never forgive myself if something were to happen." Because the "something-to-happen" could be suicide, caregivers typically cannot chance saying "no" to an overly dependent family
member's request for help. The possibility that, despite their best
efforts, someone they love might try to commit suicide fits the view
that they have no control over mental illness. However, a perceived
lack of control does not insulate caregivers from experiencing suicide attempts as a rejection of their love.

It's very upsetting to see somebody who you love . . . be completely
shut off to the world and want to not be with you—you know, want

to be gone off the face of the earth. I mean it hurts me. That is probably one of the most hurtful things I think. One time he was suicidal and I said, "Don't you even want to be here with me?" And he said, "Well I want to be here with you, but not like this."

GRADUATE STUDENT, age twenty-eight, wife

In a few cases, respondents wanted to be interviewed because a loved one had killed themselves. In the aftermath of a suicide, spouses, parents, siblings, and spouses are haunted by the feeling that were it not somehow for their neglect, the person might still be alive. A woman spoke for many when she wondered whether she might have prevented her brother's death. She said, "I knew of his illness and what he was going through, but never saw the days of real despair. . . . Now, I think. "Why didn't I just take him and say, 'Tell me what I can do to help you to get better.' . . . On the other hand, each week I go to a suicide prevention group and keep hearing the same thing; that he probably wouldn't have gotten any better. He was in as much danger of dying as somebody [with] cancer." Although it was gut-wrenching to hear the details of any suicide, the pain of children whose parents killed themselves was impossible to imagine. Clearly, though, a parent's death from suicide was an overwhelming psychological event that continues to shape the adult lives of these "children." Michelle, who, just past her sixteenth birthday, found her mother shot to death in their bathroom, worries how she will eventually explain grandma's death to her own three-year-old son. She also fears that she might be replicating her mother's life:

> It's just too much to handle sometimes, to think that Frankie is never ever going to be able to see her. You know, someday I am going to have to tell him what happened to grandma. And I am not the type of person who would lie to him. I'll tell him exactly what I am telling you with my reasoning of why she wanted to do it and everything else. I don't intend to hide anything from him, but it is not going to be an easy thing. It is not something that I want to do. And every

now and then I get afraid that he is going to think that maybe I am just like that too. You know, and I don't want him to be in the same kind of situation. I am always afraid . . . what if when he is twelve that he [becomes like] I was, coming home from school seeing me laying down on the couch watching the soaps in my robe. It gets me really upset and really depressed. So many things have happened to me that just one little memory triggers everything that has happened and then every memory is going on in my head and I can't get rid of them.

UNEMPLOYED, *age twenty-two, daughter*

Of the three Cs discussed in this chapter, it may be hardest for family members to act on the theory that they have no control over a sick person. Because we so crave a sense of order, it is impossible for a parent, spouse, child, or sibling to stand by idly as a mentally ill person wreaks havoc in their life. Realizing quickly that they have no significant control over illness itself, I have shown how family members try to impose order on the environment by adopting a managerial role. However, this strategy also poses difficulties because too much managing, by fostering dependence, may exacerbate the problem and ultimately contribute to greater disorder. While understanding the dangers of enabling, caregivers, with some exceptions, cannot withdraw their help and support. Even as they "save" an ill person from themselves, they know they might be contributing to the disorder they seek desperately to contain. It is an example of a false economy in which a short-run gain becomes the basis for a long-term loss. Because the emotional stakes in caring for someone they love are so high, family members cannot know whether it is best to work still harder at gaining control or to decrease those same efforts. It's an agonizing dilemma to be in and to have to live with.

Family members' theories about cause, cure, and control are constructed to deal with the myriad daily problems and concrete decisions posed by a partner's, child's, brother's, sister's, mother's, or father's mental illness. Because these theories are largely used to navigate the immediate, face-to-face challenges of living with an emotionally ill person, the various bureaucracies connected with mental health have so far been in the background of our conversation. Thus far, you have heard people speak only sparingly about their dealings with doctors, psychologists, hospitals, halfway houses, government agencies, and private insurance companies. In Chapter 6, caregivers' dealings with the range of institutions and people part of the mental health system will be brought to the foreground of our continuing discussion. That I have not attended to these institutions until now should not be taken as evidence of their lesser importance in the lives of the people I interviewed. To the contrary, negotiating the mental health system is surely among the most difficult, frustrating, perplexing, and anger-generating features of caregiving.

Nineteenth-century social scientists, living through the monumental social changes that accompanied industrialization and urbanization, sought to comprehend their effects on both individual behaviors and society. Max Weber was among the first to identify the essential characteristics of bureaucratic organizations.[34] Although Weber understood bureaucracies as the most efficient means for managing the business of an increasingly complex society, he worried greatly about their dehumanizing effects. Bureaucratic organizations exemplified Weber's principle of *rationalization*—the systematic and logical application of formal rules and procedures to every aspect of modern life. In his writings, he demonstrated how this principle came to permeate all spheres of life, ranging from economic activities to even art and classical music. In the final analysis, Weber remained deeply pessimistic about the prospects for a fully human life as bureaucratic policies increasingly reduced individuals to files in anonymous record-keeping systems. His prescient image of the future pictured a social world that inevitably catches all of us within the "iron cage of bureaucracy."

We all find it frustrating to cope with the red tape of bureaucracies. However, when someone becomes desperately ill and caregivers try to find the best doctors, to arrange for hospitalizations, to help an incapacitated family member apply for disability, to learn their eligibility for government benefits, and to comprehend what private insurance will cover, their dealings with bureaucracies can become maddening. The stories I heard during interviews and within the Family and Friends group reminded me of the plight of Franz Kafka's character, Joseph K., in his haunting novel, *The Trial*.[35] Like Joseph K., caregivers become ensnared in a bewildering and endless maze of paper, policies, unanswered telephone calls, inaccurate information, and, too often, insensitive bureaucrats who seem unmoved by their acute distress.

Central to sociological thinking is the idea that the dramas of daily life occur within larger historical and institutional settings. As Peter and Bridgitte Berger put it, "First of all, crucially and continuously, we inhabit the micro-world of our immediate experience with others in face-to-face relations. Beyond that, we inhabit a macro-world consisting of much larger structures and involving us in relations with others that are mostly abstract, anonymous and remote. Both worlds are essential to our experience of society, and ... each world depends upon the other for its meaning to us."[36] The character of the dialectical relationship between everyday life and the larger social forces embodied by bureaucratic institutions becomes altogether too clear when a family member becomes catastrophically ill. In trying to secure necessary health and financial resources, caregivers must figure out how a range of bureaucracies *really* function. It is an unenviable task and one that only heightens their burden. To survive a family member's illness, caregivers must also survive the mental health system. Their struggle to do that forms the substance for Chapter 6.

SIX

Surviving the System

He was in his dorm and he was obviously psychotic. I
said [to the psychiatrist], "My son is talking to a closet.
... He is obviously psychotic. Is there any way that we
can intervene at this point without waiting until he becomes totally [self-destructive]?" He says, "No, just
wait until he is in total crisis and bring him to an emergency room."

ADMINISTRATIVE ASSISTANT, *age fifty-three, mother*

I think that the mental health system is so wound up
in eight hundred million circles. . . . The circles and the
hoops you have to jump through are ridiculous.

GRADUATE STUDENT, *age twenty-eight, wife*

My interviews followed a general pattern. After a little light banter,
I told folks about the intentions of my work. I affirmed that I would
never breach their confidentiality. I also explained that they should
feel absolutely free to say if any of my questions felt "out of
bounds." Once I started taping our talk, I asked a few who-are-you
type questions about religion, occupation, age, family structure, and
the like. Ordinarily, my first substantive question asked respondents
to try recalling the very first moment it entered their consciousness
that something was wrong with their spouse, parent, sibling, or
child. Although such a global invitation normally got things going,
respondents were nevertheless tentative during the first forty-five
minutes, or so, of the interview. Understandably, they wanted to
get a better sense of my purposes, the nature of my questions, my

capacity to listen, and the authenticity of my interest. Nearly always, the conversation became freer, deeper, more spontaneous, and less self-conscious during the last two-thirds of our talk.

Nearly from the moment we met, I felt comfortable with Carol. She had an engaging demeanor, laughed easily, was clearly glad for the opportunity to tell her story, and responded openly to my question about the start of her daughter's trouble. As our conversation moved along, Carol also freely expressed hurt, anger, frustration, and confusion about "the year from hell" caused by Jeanne's manic-depression. As with nearly every interview, Carol wanted to talk about the particular illness-connected issues that she found especially oppressive. Thus, our conversation turned to money matters. Carol then produced a letter she wanted me to have. She explained that her daughter is without health insurance, that, together, they "are in the process of appealing" the state's refusal to grant her disability status. Carol explained that she constructed the letter with the hope that someone—*anyone*—in the state system would finally understand Jeanne's needs. The letter, she told me, "is an insurance story, but it is also really an overview of the last eight or ten years with my daughter."

Carol's letter was addressed "to whom it may concern" because, after countless telephone calls she remained "totally baffled by the process. Totally baffled." Her plan was to send the letter to whomever she could identify in the health system who might somehow be in a position to provide guidance. She wanted me to have the letter, both because it offered a history of her daughter's illness and because it reflected her own confusion, frustration, and anger toward a bureaucratic health system that she simply could not understand, a system that seemed unable to comprehend the seriousness of her daughter's illness, if it was not altogether indifferent to her needs. The letter artfully detailed the contours of both Jeanne's illness and Carol's attempts to secure health insurance. It told how both Jeanne's health and insurance problems picked up momentum when she turned nineteen, went off to Nicaragua, had a full-blown manic episode, was hospitalized for a time, came home for a while, and then "took off . . . to get a job on a fishing boat." No longer

covered by her own health insurance, Carol found, after many fruitless attempts, that private insurance companies would not issue
Jeanne a policy because of the prior hospitalization.

Having received a diagnosis of manic-depressive illness did little
to stop the downward spiral of Jeanne's life. At about the time she
returned home, "she went off her medication and the year from
hell began." The letter detailed how in that year Jeanne owned three
different cars, had two car accidents, and received multiple speeding
tickets. She also was arrested for assault and battery, was obliged
to make three court appearances, "lost control of money and
bounced several checks," and in the following spring "crashed and
made her first suicide attempt." In the middle of the year, Jeanne
"was permanently denied any mental health coverage." Carol's letter further detailed, "When I asked for an explanation, I was told
that she would need to demonstrate that she was healthy by going
off her medication. My attempt to explain that being *on* medication
is the best way to promote good mental health was disregarded. I
was appalled to discover the ignorance and misunderstanding that
surrounds mental illness." The letter continues:

> I worry about the consequences of no insurance, but I can't imagine
> how, other than CommonHealth [the state system], she will ever be
> insured. Although she is an extraordinary nanny, she has been un-
> able to hold other jobs for more than a few months. She was fired
> as a security guard because she was constantly late; she was fired as
> a waitress because she became belligerent over scheduling; she was
> fired as a maid because she was disorganized and uncooperative; she
> had a verbal disagreement with the owner of a sub shop and quit.
> It has been very hard for me to watch her fail so often. . . . Jeanne
> is a very fragile young woman. I think she should qualify for [state]
> medical assistance.

The letter then concludes with this paragraph:

> As I wade through this process, I'm sure I will learn how the insur-
> ance system "works," but for now I feel baffled. . . . I haven't been

able to find anyone to help me. If this letter has fallen into your hands, by chance or on purpose, and if you can help me to understand how to successfully help my daughter to negotiate her way through this medical assistance process, *please* do.

Carol's letter centers on the intricacies of getting insurance for a mentally ill person. Unfortunately, the difficulties detailed in her letter and in our conversation were typical. Everyone must navigate a maze of rules and regulations, confusing paperwork, and the sometimes dozens of hours of phoning that accompanies efforts to secure private or government insurance. Although discussed in nearly every interview, figuring out the rules of the insurance game is only one of the bureaucratic tasks caregivers confront. In addition, they typically must learn how to deal with the local police, community crisis teams, the court system, psychiatric hospitals, doctors, therapists of all sorts, and community outpatient services. Taken together, these organizations and the people who compose them constitute the mental health "system"—a complex network of bureaucracies that absolutely no one finds "user-friendly." Every person interviewed expressed anger, frustration, and confusion about the twin difficulties of getting the right care for a family member and finding ways to pay for it. In the pages that follow, I describe what it is like for family caregivers to deal with the range of institutions that presumably exist to provide quality care for the mentally ill but, ironically, often seem instead an obstacle to just that goal.

In the broadest sense, this chapter conforms closely to the most essential concerns of my discipline. It might properly be said that sociology is the study of how social structures structure us. Among all the social science disciplines, sociology is most resolutely focused on how our "social location" within an intersecting system of groups, organizations, and institutions shape our options, our behaviors, and our perspectives about the world. A sociological perspective looks at the ways that all of our lives are shaped by external forces over which we often have little control. As in other chapters,

I will be highlighting the particular contingencies experienced in getting help for mental illness. However, the stories you will hear reflect the sorts of problems faced by Americans with all kinds of health problems who are not well served by an increasingly complex, sometimes incomprehensible health system that is pushed along by bureaucratic logic and economic constraints instead of the well-being of human beings.[1]

Systems often operate in a paradoxical fashion.[2] Here the paradox is that while every element of the system presumably seeks the same general goal (the health of ill people), the "cultures" of mental health bureaucrats, doctors, and family caregivers intersect in a fashion that often undermines that goal. You might think of bureaucrats, patients, professional healers, and family members as each speaking different dialects of the same language. Because each actor in the bureaucratic play comes from a "different place," with his or her own distinctive concerns, rules, values, and knowledge, the likelihood of miscommunication and frustrating experiences is heightened. My goal in this chapter is to illustrate how the different interests, perspectives, and system stakes held by patients, caregivers, health professionals, and administrators generate tremendous caregiver frustration. To see how this is so, I will organize this chapter in terms of the sequencing of system experiences as they normally occur in the unfolding of a family member's illness.

The "institutional careers" of both patients and family caregivers begin with a crisis.[3] Somewhere along the line there is no denying that something is dreadfully wrong and that an ill person desperately needs help. Sometimes the crisis unfolds gradually enough for family members to seek therapy discretely. More usually, the first crisis is both dramatic and severe enough that family caregivers quickly learn about community crisis teams and the laws governing involuntary commitment. At some point, every ill family member entered a hospital. Hospitalization is a pivotal moment in the joint institutional history of caregivers and patients. Once in the hospital, family members also enter the professional domain of psychiatrists and other mental health professionals. By now, caregivers must also find an answer to the bottom-line question, "Who is going to pay for the care?" Thus, every caregiver eventually faced four generic system-related tasks, roughly in this order:

1. MANAGING CRISIS
2. HOSPITALIZATION
3. DEALING WITH DOCTORS
4. PAYING FOR CARE

Each time ill people and their family caregivers find themselves dealing with a different part of the mental health system they have, in effect, entered a new cultural world. In this way, caregivers are rather like travelers visiting a series of foreign countries, each with its distinctive habits, regulations, norms, and beliefs. As they make their way through the several institutional stops on their mental health itinerary, they must somehow quickly learn each country's language and culture. Caregivers quickly realize that each part of the bureaucratic network operates in terms of a set of requirements that typically do not fit well with their own needs, concerns, and anxieties. Rather than minimizing their pain, encounters with the system too often exacerbate their troubles.

Managing Crisis

In Chapter 3, on the emotions that surround the onset of mental illness, I described caregivers as suffering from "emotional anomie." I meant to convey with this concept that caregivers are stunned by the events surrounding the first dramatic episode of mental illness and simply don't know what to feel. I borrow the term anomie from the work of several social theorists who have used it to depict a state of "normlessness."[4] First used to describe the kind of bewilderment that accompanies rapid social change, the French sociologist Emile Durkheim linked the effects of normlessness to rates of suicide.[5] When mental illness makes its first dramatic appearance, caregivers are thrust into a kind of surreal world where nothing makes sense. At first they don't know what to do, how to proceed, or whom to rely on.

> We knew right then [that] we needed help. So, the next day I went to work. I was like numb, but I went to work. I didn't know where to turn. I didn't go to anyone at work first. I didn't know who to call. It didn't occur to me to look in the Yellow Pages and call a Counseling Center. What I did was call the Department of Mental Health . . . and I left this, like, urgent message with a secretary that I needed to talk to someone, that we were having a crisis. And she told me that someone would call me right back. Well, I never got a call. And I thought, "Well, so much for the Department of Mental Health."
>
> SECRETARY, *age fifty-one, mother*

↩

> I walked into Mass Mental Health . . . and I went in and I am like, "I need help." I was like, "I don't know what kind of help. I don't know. I'm open to anything."
>
> STUDENT, *age twenty-five, wife*

↩

> It was before I put him in the hospital. I called this therapist and said, "I gotta do something." And he said, "I can't do anything." I said, "You can't? You know, he stopped taking his medication. He's terrible. You've got to do something! He can't exist like this." And he said, "I can't do anything." He wasn't willing to do anything at all. . . . He didn't appreciate the severity of his [her husband's] depression, I think.
>
> HOMEMAKER, *age fifty-two, spouse*

Bureaucratic systems normalize, routinize, and rationalize as usual the events that caregivers are experiencing as a terrorizing crisis. Such an observation extends to all professionals who deal routinely with events that carry tremendous significance for their clients. To the doctor conducting the operation, it's just another day's work. In the same way, members of crisis teams, ambulance drivers, policemen, nurses, and health administrators deal with other people's crises on a daily basis. What family members experience as dramatic and chaotic turmoil, they experience as routine, even boring. Perhaps family members can understand such a demeanor in retrospect, but in the middle of their crisis with a family member, the contrast between their own feelings and those who come to help is utterly jarring. Initial contacts with police and crisis teams are a preview of the sort of "bureaucratization" of their personal problem that will eventually characterize their relations with all sorts of "officials" and professionals. Although caregivers might understand the need for it, the ritualization of their crisis feels callous to them. Here's how the police handled one crisis:

> I see a police car go flying by her [neighbor's] house. . . . I knew that the Counseling Center had sent the police. . . . And, this is so incredible to me. I mean, they would have taken him there, right then and there, except it would have been like arresting him for damaging property, or something. And I said to them, I couldn't do it. I said to them, "Just go in and talk to him"—we're out on the driveway. So silly, you know, talk to him! The cops, that was fine with them, you know. So they go into the house and Mike's sitting there. He doesn't look crazy. He looks like he's fine, you know? And I had cleaned up everything he had broken. There was no evidence of the stuff he'd been smashing. . . . You know, all this broken stuff, I'd cleaned it up, put it in the trash; there was no evidence that anything had been wrong. So they said, "Mike, we hear that things have been a little tense around here, and you've been breaking some things," or whatever. . . . And in the meantime, one of the police officers . . . there was a novel sitting on the coffee table. And he looks at the novel and says to me, "Oh, are you reading that? Is that a good book?" I'm thinking, "Oh———," you know?
>
> SECRETARY, *age fifty-one, mother*

Although the emphasis of this discussion is on the institutional history that begins with the first dramatic crisis in a family, it is not surprising that over time caregivers become "veterans" who learn to handle succeeding crises with something approaching the attitude of mental health professionals. As they eventually come to understand the culture of the mental health system and then deal with repeated episodes, they too learn to routinize the procedures necessary to have someone removed from the home, to get into a hospital, to get to the correct emergency room, and the like. It is slightly ironic that caregivers eventually replicate the sort of distanced or removed behaviors of those who daily deal with crisis; they come to adopt the same kind of cool, business-like demeanor that previously felt objectionable when first witnessed in others.

The first time you experience [a crisis], you know . . . you are having all these [feelings]. I mean, you may have a heart attack, you don't know what is going on. You go into this [place], it's like a prison. You have doors that lock behind you. It's all locked up. You have keys to get in there and then Adam goes in, and he told me, "Get the fuck out of his room." . . . I was . . . in such shock and numb, but you don't cry because you just, you need to take care of things. . . . He was there for four weeks, for that first incident . . . But the thing is now that I'm experienced, that wouldn't bother me. . . . Well, now, so what if he has schizophrenia? You know, just how is he? I mean, I'm immune to this.

ADMINISTRATIVE ASSISTANT, *age fifty-three, mother*

⌣

I think time has taught me that this is something that we're going to live with. Maybe you go a year, maybe two years. I think I have enough support systems in place at this stage of the game that I would get immediate intervention. And I've learned that. And I've learned how to do that. And I think I have enough of a support system at this stage that I can do that. Whereas, I didn't before.

SALESPERSON, *age thirty-five, wife*

When persons are so sick that community crisis teams are called in, the decision is frequently made on the spot that they must be hospitalized, typically against their will. As several stories in earlier chapters illustrate, seeing a loved one removed from their home, sometimes in handcuffs, is traumatic for caregiving novices. It is terrible to feel that you have somehow betrayed a family member. The only comfort in seeing a child, spouse, sibling, or parent "taken away" is the expectation that they will be getting the treatment they need, that families will have a respite from the turmoil of madness, and that the ill person will finally have asylum. Although they can't appreciate it at the time, caregivers may be fortunate that a family member is so obviously and desperately ill that there is no question about the need to hospitalize them. In other cases caregivers learn that psychosis alone is not enough to guarantee admission to a hospital. Discovering that a clearly psychotic person is not yet sufficiently sick to receive treatment is often caregivers' first brutal hint that they face a system whose regulations are inimicable to mentally ill people and their families.

The complexities, paradoxes, ironies, and confusion in getting care are massively compounded in the case of mental illness. Caregivers who don't know the laws in Massachusetts where this study was conducted are typically shocked to learn that the health system operates with two standards—one for people suffering from physical illnesses and a second for the mentally ill. The problem arises because mentally ill people often cannot recognize that they are sick and do not wish to be helped. Thereby, the case of mental illness routinely raises human rights issues that rarely enter into decisions about treating people with other acute illnesses. In Massachusetts, as in many states, mentally ill people cannot be hospitalized against their will until it has been clearly determined that they are a danger to themselves or to other people.[6] It frequently shocks family caregivers that they cannot get a person hospitalized when the severity of their illness seems so transparently clear. In the middle of a family crisis, debates about the "rights" of the mentally ill seem irrelevant. To be told that someone so obviously ill will not be allowed into the system seems itself, in the moment of crisis, a form of institutional insanity.

They're too sick to realize that they're sick. That's one of the things that's so frustrating about mental illness is that the person that's making the judgment can't make the judgment. And so, right now she won't go to the hospital. She's paranoid. The only way she goes in the hospital is if she does something that seems like she's sick enough, a danger to herself. . . . You could bring her to the hospital three nights in a row, get three different professionals, and one will commit her, but two won't. So it's a frustrating system. . . . She can open a car door in the middle of driving down the road [to the hospital], but she's not committable.

ACCOUNTANT, *age thirty-five, daughter*

↜

I tried to get her into the hospital and I couldn't. And there was a little pip-squeak shrink in the ER, you know, one of the resident types, and he was relatively decent, but there I am sobbing my guts out, sobbing, sobbing, sobbing, trying to get this kid into the hospital because she is not safe, but she is also not crazy. She is not committable.

PHYSICAL THERAPIST, *age forty-nine, mother*

↜

I am a basket case [at this point]. I went to the local hospital and they sent down the doctor on call. She was a sweetheart. She was probably thirty years old. She said, "Do you want to talk?" I told her all of these things about Andy, what we had been through. She said, "I just wish you the best of luck trying to get him in [the hospital]." She didn't have a solution. . . . I asked her if she did private practice, you know. She doesn't, so anyway, from that I thought, "How am I going to get him in? How am I going to do this?" I spent eight hours on the phone one Saturday and guess what, nobody could help me. It was like, they couldn't do this unless this, this and that.

REAL ESTATE BROKER, age forty-four, mother

In the middle of a crisis, especially the first one, as they experience the absolute turmoil wrought by mental illness, caregivers have one aim—to get their sick family member into the system. Admission to a mental hospital solves the initial crisis and provides some relief. One mother of a seriously suicidal daughter said that "before she went into the hospital, twenty-four hours a day I was awake. I never slept at night. When she rolled over in that bed I heard her." Similarly, a woman caring for her sister said, "When you get to that point [of crisis] and someone is hospitalized, it is traumatic, but it is also a relief." And another parent, although greatly pained by having to commit her daughter, felt liberated by the decision. She told me:

> We did section 12 her the first time in July and I said, "Oh my God, will my kid ever forgive me?" And the therapist said, "Someday she'll forgive you." And I brought her in on the fourth of July and they weren't sure if they were going to keep her or not so they called [*names psychiatrist*] and he said, "Keep her." She looked at me and she said, with hate in her eyes, "You get me out of here." And I said, "No way am I getting you out of here. You need to be here." And she said, "If you don't let me out of here, you will never see me again." And I said, "If I get you out of here, I may never see you again." And I walked out the door with a thousand pounds off my shoulders because she was safe and they kept her there the whole weekend. Oh my God, it was the first peaceful weekend I've had in years because she wasn't on the streets. . . . She was safe.

PHYSICAL THERAPIST, age forty-nine, mother

Once an ill person is hospitalized, caregivers feel relief that their immediate role in controlling a bewildering crisis has ended. Admission to the hospital feels like a victory, and those new to the caregiving process expect that professionals will shortly solve the problem that precipitated the hospitalization. They are soon disabused of this idea. Hospitalization is simply the starting point for a series of continuing problems, many of them arising from an inability to "work" the system that is supposed to be working for them. Hospitalization they soon discover is just the beginning of an institutional journey for which they are ill prepared.

Hospitalization

Initial episodes of mental illness are completely bewildering to family members because, although they know that something is desperately wrong, they have no clear idea what to call it, what has caused it, how long it's likely to last, what treatments will be like, whether medications will help, and so on. Once they are past the immediate crisis preceding hospitalization, caregivers expect that doctors, nurses, social workers, and other mental health experts will clear up their confusion, that after the ill person is properly evaluated, all their questions will shortly be answered. Instead, they confront the unsettling truth that hospitalization often settles little. Rather than gaining greater clarity into the situation of their ill family members, caregivers bitterly complained to me that they were kept in the dark; no one seemed willing to tell them much of anything. They craved and expected information. Instead, they experienced a system that disregarded, marginalized, and treated them as though they were simply disinterested onlookers to a roadside tragedy. For reasons they couldn't comprehend, those in charge were unwilling to share much information at all.

> And so, we didn't know what this was going to be [like]. [I wish] somebody had just talked to us about the reason they were doing what they were doing and what was the effect of the medication they were going to give him. Just give us information, like information was what we didn't have. We were just ignorant. So, in that setting

[hospital] we learned very little really about mental health, mental conditions, mental treatment, even though Eileen [wife] was, I think, comforted that lithium was a natural salt. . . . There was sort of the feeling, "Look, we have a patient. Our priorities are the patient. We do not have the staff, the facility, and so on, to deal with you people—You know, to educate you."

RETIRED SCHOOLTEACHER, *age sixty-two, father*

〜

So anyway, she got [admitted], I think it was on a Tuesday. By Friday I had still not met with anybody in the hospital to talk about her care, her course of treatment, nothing. I was ripshit because I am a really involved mother and they haven't told me anything about her.

PHYSICAL THERAPIST, *age forty-nine, mother*

〜

We didn't have that much support, I don't think, when he was first hospitalized as far as information. I don't think that we knew the course that his illness would take. His first illness, he was hospitalized a good three weeks anyway. And if I remember, we had one family meeting at the hospital which was a complete disaster. I mean . . . our family ended up not speaking to each other and got very little information.

TECHNOLOGY LICENSER, *age thirty-three, sister*

〜

At [*names hospital*] they would not let me see her the first time she was there and I found that extremely angering because when you're in their office, their lovely office, they give you all this crap about family involvement. And I couldn't even get her social worker to call me on the phone. And the only time I could talk to her was on a pay phone. What is that? That's just lousy. And I really feel like it was because she is on state aid.

ARTIST, *age forty-four, partner*

The last respondent raises a question about the relationship between quality of health care and one's capacity to pay. The continuing unpleasant reality is that, for those requiring long-term treatment in state mental health facilities, hospital conditions are sometimes awful. The history of deinstitutionalization of mental patients is by now well documented.[7] Part of the urge toward deinstitutionalization, made possible by the discovery of relatively effective antipsychotic drugs, was the horrible, dehumanizing circumstances of those confined to state hospitals. While it would, of course, be unfair to lump together all state-run mental health facilities, several of those interviewed were horrified by the deplorable conditions in the places their family members were obliged to go for "treatment." Here, at some length, is one person's description of the conditions at a state hospital, a description of the sort I heard from too many others without the money for long-term private care:

When he first went there, he was on a locked ward there for a few months. It's like prison. It's like going to prison. . . . I was warned that the locked unit at [*names hospital*] is behind probably a twenty-foot high chain link fence, a good fifteen to twenty feet high. You have to be buzzed in by the DMH [Department of Mental Health] police. It's like going to jail. And the locked building is at the very end of the campus. So, first of all you're driving through what you could tell was once very beautiful, but there are all these boarded-up buildings. The roads are just in terrible shape, chunks of pavement missing, and potholes. It's just in total disrepair. And then you drive up to these big gates. First you have to get a pass. They call ahead and tell them that you're coming. And then you come to these gates and you have to press a buzzer. And there are cameras on you, so they can see who is there. And they buzz you in. And then they have to unlock a door to let you in. Then you have to sign in. You know, all of these security procedures. . . . It just looked so dreary to me. . . . I just found it very depressing. And the patients that I saw there I found very depressing. . . . I guess I'm just not used to the public mental health system, but it's so depressing that I cannot see how anyone can get well there.

You know, my son has this terrible, terrible mental illness, but he's still got this good mind. He wants to read; he wants to learn. . . . He's on this floor . . . this is what I see. I see this old woman without teeth, babbling, babbling, babbling about three young women whose husbands got killed, and all these millions of dollars got stolen. She's just babbling, on and on about this. Then there is an old man, sitting in the chair. And he's sitting there, looking at this old lady and he goes, "Are you accusing me of killing my parents?" And then, there is this other toothless woman who is screaming and swearing at the mental health workers. And there is my son, who has done some terrible things and is very ill, yes. He's just standing there, waiting to get his medication. And he's just standing there, amidst all of this. . . . "I'm sorry," I said to the staff, "I know you can only work with what you've got, but that building is so depressing. How can anyone get well?"

SECRETARY, *age fifty-one, mother*

It does not take caregivers long to develop a cynicism about the hospital system. In the worst instances, caregivers were shocked and frightened by the context of the hospital, places altogether too reminiscent of the "snakepits" that motivated the social reforms intended by the deinstitutionalization movement. However, even in those hospitals where their children, spouses, parents, or siblings were well treated, family members were normally left out of the informational loop. Sometimes, it was the legal requirement to protect the confidentiality of patients older than eighteen that kept them uninformed. Although such regulations make sense in the abstract, they form the basis for yet another caregiving paradox in the case of mental illness. Maintaining the confidentiality of adults seems sensible only when patients can make reasoned judgments about sharing the details of their medical condition with family caregivers.

Legal requirements aside, it appears contrary to the culture of the mental hospitals to be attentive to the concerns, fears, and confusion of family members who are totally dazed by the sequence of events that eventuated in a family member's hospitalization. While feeling generally shut out, lost, disconnected, confused, and angered by their nonrole in the treatment of a loved one, caregivers expected to at least leave the hospital with some clarity about the problem. At the very least, they hoped that someone would give them a diagnosis and a prognosis of a family member's condition. What they generally discovered, early in another person's illness history, is that neither a cure nor a firm diagnosis would be forthcoming. One person spoke for several whose expectations for even minimal information were not met when she said, "I don't remember hospitalization being a great help or answering questions. I felt that I couldn't get any answers. I guess you always expect there to be some sort of diagnostic resolution, at least." It may, in fact, take years to get a firm diagnosis. Sometimes, family members eventually learn of the diagnosis accidentally.

> No one talked to us. No professionals ever talked with us. . . . None of these people talked to us. We didn't really know what was going on. We would just know she was being admitted to the hospital. We would visit her. But no one would ever give you a call and talk to you about a diagnosis or anything. The only reason I [eventually] found out she had been diagnosed as schizophrenic, was because I found a paper in her room . . . that described it when she was in the hospital.
>
> ACCOUNTANT, *age thirty-five, daughter*

↩

> I think about two or three years ago she started taking Clozaril. . . . I was talking to a psychiatrist two years ago, and I said, "I'm not sure what she has," and [then] I said, "she takes this drug." And he says, "Well that is for schizophrenia."
>
> INSURANCE ADMINISTRATOR, *age forty-six, daughter*

In more than one case, family members came, over a period of years, to doubt the validity of the whole diagnostic process in the matter of mental illness. One exceedingly articulate fellow, who had been dealing with a chronically schizophrenic mother since early childhood, offered a critique of the medical model when applied to psychiatric disorders. His assessment parallels many published accounts also claiming psychiatric disorders to be political and cultural designations, not purely scientific judgments.[8]

> I understand that if you are a Western doctor or you believe the Western model, that the point of diagnosis is treatment, so that you can treat someone better. But if the person gets a diagnosis and the treatment is not applicable, then what is the point; what is the use? And that seems to be the constant problem of mental illness . . . with schizophrenia, bipolar disorder, with depression, with borderline personality. There is, you know, the DSM, this huge manual of diagnosis, and yet there isn't a great percentage of people who seem to benefit by it in my opinion.
>
> ARTIST, *age thirty, son*

Years ago, the sociologists Everett Hughes, Howard Becker, and Blanche Geer studied how medical students were eventually made into doctors.[9] A central thread in their description of the process was what they called "the fate of idealism." Over time, doctors-to-be must give up their initially idealistic ideas about practicing medicine in order to function in the day-to-day world of hospital life. Analogously, patients and their families, especially those initially unfamiliar with the mental health system, suffer a negative fate of idealism. They are caught in a terrible double bind. Someone they love is too ill to remain at home and so they are relieved when, sometimes after much wrangling and torment, they are finally admitted to a hospital. It doesn't take long, though, to realize that hospitalization is, at best, a stopgap measure. Some quickly become skeptical, if not downright cynical, about the mental health system. They are particularly shocked to learn that a suffering family member often remains hospitalized only as long as insurance covers their stay. When their insurance runs out, patients are put out. It's hard not to begin resenting a system so transparently guided by bureaucratic imperatives.

In the most recent meetings at the hospital—in the meetings where my brother is manic—they are just looking at us in the face and saying, "Well if he doesn't take his medicine we are going to release him and if he murders somebody he murders somebody." So, you know . . . with the shorter insurance days and lack of medical insurance and this that and the other thing, I mean, what this doctor was essentially saying is that if your brother doesn't comply within the next twenty-four hours to take lithium, we are going to release him, manic or not. To a family member that is absolutely frightening. They just can't imagine the impact that has on people sitting in the room who, you know, have watched my brother threaten to kill people, threaten to kill himself.

TECHNOLOGY LICENSER, age thirty-three, sister

↩

He did [finally] get a diagnosis of paranoid schizophrenia, which I felt was more accurate than depression. So, we said, "Mike cannot come home." You know, it was more for our kids than for us, but it was for all of us. I said, "He can't come home." Well, there was no housing available, and Mike was to be discharged into a homeless shelter. Honest to God, they really do that. I thought they were joking. I said, "Well, if he goes to a homeless shelter, he'll die. Either he will die, or someone else will die. He won't take his medication. He'll become psychotic. He'll be homeless. Either he will die on the street, or someone else is going to die." "Well, that's where he is to go. He's going to be discharged to a homeless shelter." So, of course, we said, "Well then, he'll come home." And once you say that, that's it.

SECRETARY, age fifty-one, mother

↩

And when they even talk about insurance, you feel like going after somebody's throat. You feel like saying, "This is my son, this isn't a friggin' dollar sign."

REAL ESTATE BROKER, *age forty-four, mother*

Insurance "horror stories" were unfortunately common. In one case, after three weeks of maneuvering, a woman was able to arrange for her husband, recently released from the hospital after a course of electroconvulsive shock treatments, to attend a hospital's day treatment program. Each morning for more than a month she dropped him off at the treatment center. Things were going well enough until she received a distraught telephone call from her husband who had been "kicked out" of the program. Here's what happened:

They had had some neurological consults set up for him and then one day he just called me at work and left a message that said, "Hey, I am standing outside of [names hospital]. They said I can't come here any more. Please come get me." Unfortunately it was at a time when I had [just] gone into a meeting. I obviously left the meeting when I got the message and I went to get him and he was just in such a horrendous state. It was freezing outside. It was either January or December. . . . I remember he was wearing his winter coat and it was cold and, I said, "What happened?" [He said] "I don't know. They just said my money ran out and I couldn't stay any more and that they had gotten a message on Friday and it was a Monday and that they didn't have any way to get in touch with us over the weekend." So I managed to get him to go back inside. . . . I managed to get him to at least come in and sit down and talk with me about it there because I wanted to go talk to somebody. But he was in such a state that he would not let me leave him. . . . He was just like, "NO, I just want to go home. Please take me home." So we get him home and . . . I called every single resource I had. I called his doctor. I called his psychotherapist. I called the insurance company. . . . I left a really nasty message on the insurance's machine that basically said,

"If my husband kills himself or has to go into the hospital for doing
so, I will sue you for everything that you possibly can imagine."
That was just a burst [of anger] but it was a serious burst because
I meant it. I was really hurt by what they did.

STUDENT, *age twenty-eight, spouse*

Dealing with Doctors

Some years ago, the sociologist Eliot Freidson commented that "the
relationship of the expert to modern life seems in fact to be one of
the central problems of our time, for at its heart lie the issue of
democracy and freedom and the degree to which [people] can
shape the character of their own lives."[10] Similarly, writers like
Philip Rieff have maintained that a kind of "therapeutic culture"
has triumphed in the United States, characterized by the ascendancy
of the professions, medical professionals in particular.[11] The historian Christopher Lasch has also written extensively about the burgeoning role of experts in shaping our self-images.[12] Lasch maintains that professional experts are increasingly intruding into family
life, once a private oasis in an otherwise public world. He argues
that through the "colonizing" efforts of therapeutic experts, the
family has increasingly come under the close scrutiny of the state.

Lasch argues that the therapeutic state composed of doctors, psychiatrists, guidance counselors, child development specialists, and
the like has not arisen simply through the impersonal workings of
historical forces. He reads these developments as part of a political
process of social control. His interpretation of nineteenth-century
history is that the rise of the therapeutic professions exposed the
family to a system of social control based on systematic observation
and surveillance. By bringing sexuality, childrearing, and other family practices under ceaseless technocratic intervention, professionals
simultaneously wrested control over domestic life from the family
itself. In this respect, Lasch interprets the rise of the therapeutic
state as a political event that allowed greater bureaucratic control
over any dangerous socialistic energies that an unsupervised family

structure might potentially create. According to these views, Sigmund Freud is one of the great stabilizers of liberal capitalism because his ideas gave rise to a psychiatric apparatus that governs society by prescribing the standards that define normality.

> Doctors, criminologists . . . and other members of the learned professions to which in the twentieth century were added social workers, psychiatrists, educators, marriage counselors, child development experts, pediatricians, parole officers, judges of the juvenile courts, in short the modern apparatus of resocialization—governed society not "by right but by teaching technique, not by law but by normalization, not by punishment but by control."[13]

Whether or not we agree with Lasch's political interpretation of history, one thing is clear. The development of a society that is highly dependent on experts of all sorts, but particularly therapeutic experts who have come to define the normative boundaries of our daily lives, is unique in human history. Along with Freidson, Rieff, and Lasch, I consider this an historical development having powerful consequences for the general ordering of society and for virtually every aspect of our daily lives. Still, however much our daily lives are shaped by experts, their role in our fates becomes dramatically magnified when a life trouble causes us to seek them out, ask for their help, and come to believe that our future well-being is in their hands. Such is certainly the case for caregivers and their ill family members who have entered the medical system, the home ballpark, as it were, of psychiatric experts. One initial surprise is the relative inaccessibility of psychiatrists, the "high priests" of the mental hospital.

> It's surprising to me the small role that psychiatrists often play in all of this. The psychiatrist had little to do with him [son]. . . . You seem to very rarely speak to a psychiatrist.
>
> SECRETARY, *age fifty-one, mother*

⌐

There were so many times that my brother was just so over-medicated, and with all the side effects. It's just a general impression I had . . . when I would visit him in the hospital. I was very upset with a lot of them [doctors]. I mean, there were one or two of them that he liked, but they ended up moving, or for one reason or another they were no longer able to treat him. I mean, they treated him well, the nurses and the staff. I think they cared. But I think the doctors that treated him didn't spend much time with him. They just kind of medicate and, you know, walk away.

ARTIST, *age thirty, brother*

If doctors are generally unavailable to their patients in mental hospitals, they are even more inaccessible to their family caregivers. Despite the fact that their patients will eventually return to their family's home, doctors once again left caregivers out of the informational loop. It seems like an odd kind of myopia on the part of mental health professionals, especially doctors. At best, family members are in doctors' peripheral vision. Their therapeutic model is of a two-person social system only—doctor and patient. Here again, we witness the contradiction that despite their centrality in the care of patients, family caregivers are typically cast to the margins of informational networks within the health system. One of the few studies to examine doctor/patient interaction with caregivers present shows that the presence of a third party, in fact, "poses serious challenges for the physician in terms of how to allocate attention."[14] Contests for the attention of physicians arise because caregivers have such strong needs to voice their own caregiving concerns and problems. The authors conclude that "because caregivers can help physicians to understand . . . patients more fully, it is imperative to utilize their knowledge . . . while maintaining patients' autonomy."[15]

Over the course of writing two books on mental illness, I have been struck by the ill feelings that patients and caregivers have about psychiatrists. In all my conversations, the relative proportion of negative to positive comments about psychiatrists among caregivers is hugely weighted toward the negative. Although I heard a few stories about marvelous psychiatrists who were seen as saviors, I much more frequently heard caregivers complain about doctors who were unwilling to listen to what they had to say, who radically decontextualized things in a way that defied common sense, who were prone to snap judgments that seemed odd and uninformed, who were callous in their comments and demeanor, and who were sometimes cavalier in blaming caregivers for the problem. Listen to what makes caregivers angry about psychiatrists. First, psychiatrists are *frequently seen as unwilling to listen* to what caregivers have to say:

> We had this collection of doctors and social workers of all sorts staring at us because we were trying to explain what had happened, but nobody was really interested in what we had to say because we were not the patient. . . . So, we tried to explain what had happened and our concerns about what was going on. We knew that his mind was under attack and had been altered, but we did not know how or why or what-have-you. . . . So, there was a lot of resistance [to talking with us]. She [social worker] just wanted to get the facts and kept saying that this is not going to be a therapy session and you have to talk to the doctor. Well, the doctor didn't want to talk to us. Nobody really wanted to talk to us.
>
> RETIRED SCHOOLTEACHER, *age sixty-two, father*

Psychiatrists frequently decontexualize their treatment by disregarding the knowledge and needs of caregivers:

> If a professional person told me that for the benefit of John [son] that I needed to change one more thing, I would just go out of my mind. . . . And it seems insane to me . . . that they will treat him, but they are only getting one side of what is really going on. . . . I have reservations about that. You know, of going in and everybody seeing

John as the person that is bipolar, has all these problems, and let's all fix everything so that life is easier for John. And if we have no stress for John, then life is perfect. Well, the real world isn't like that. And in order for me to make a stress-free world for John, that means I am shouldering even more than I need to and I don't think sometimes that people always see that, you know? Professionals get annoyed with me trying to be a part of it and yet I'm the one they are giving [the problem] back to.

HOME HEALTH AIDE, *age forty-four, mother*

Psychiatrists frequently make snap judgments without much background information:

I was really angry at the psychiatrist Monday night. He's never met any of us and he said to me, "You all should be in family counseling." And I wanted to say, "How the hell do you know this? How do you?" How dare he say we need family counseling. What does he know?

PHYSICAL THERAPIST, *age forty-nine, mother*

Psychiatrists frequently behave callously in a way that increases the caregivers' pain:

After my mom killed herself we went to a psychiatrist. It was Michelle's [sister's] idea. We went and talked to this guy and I went in and I didn't say anything. I was just going to give him his chance and see what he had to say. My sister sat down and just poured her heart out. I mean, for my sister, this is major. . . . This was a big step for her to go and talk about her feelings, you know? She told everything to this guy and he turned around and was like, "I know how you feel. I had an AIDS patient who just died a few days ago . . ." And . . . me and Michelle are just looking at him like, "Our mom just blew her brains out." You know, we are real sorry about your

AIDS patient, but they are not your family and certainly not your
mother. You know, how can you compare these two, you know?

UNEMPLOYED, age twenty-two, daughter

Psychiatrists frequently are quick to blame caregivers for their family
member's problem:

Psychiatrists. Oh, they were awful. Have you ever talked with psychiatrists? They beat my brains in. The mother. It's all her fault.

UNEMPLOYED, age fifty, mother

Before this appears to be a lopsided exercise in doctor bashing,
I should say that several respondents told of eventually finding the
"right" doctor. A mother was grateful for finding a psychiatrist
whom she refers to as "St. David" because he "gets the big picture
and a sense of what's going on." St. David was further applauded
for "being a real person." A spouse approved of her husband's
doctor who "doesn't just give him meds." A mother whose son was
diagnosed with manic-depression at age eight was grateful for a
doctor "who was just enjoying Andrew like a really nice person
would." After "going through a whole slew of them," a couple
found a "good one" who "when we go to talk with him, he'll share
his experiences. He's not just somebody sitting there with a clock
ticking and saying, 'Okay, give me your money.'" Yet another respondent appreciated a "therapist who interacts with you as a human being."

When they describe doctors as good and caring people who "interact with you as a human being," respondents imply that, as with
their own caregiving, healing practitioners are fully effective only
when their care has a loving dimension. Lauren Slater, therapist
and author, observes that psychotherapy works because of the
"love" that develops between doctor and patient.[16] And St. David's
client, quoted above, made exactly the same point in a letter to me
after reading a draft version of this book. She wrote: "The good
doctors are able to practice not just the science but the art of med-

icine. They listen and look carefully with no preconceived ideas or stereotypes. They see and hear not just what is said and done, but how it 'feels.' They have well-tuned emotional antennae. They also care deeply and are able to show that they care. . . . It is also important to note that they not only take care of the primary patient, but the whole family. In your book you state many times how families take care of the ill member out of love, how they make incredible sacrifices out of love. The good care providers also act out of love and have an equally powerful commitment to care."

Comments about "good" doctors are revealing because they help to illuminate contradictions between the needs of "clients" and the contemporary organization of professional work.[17] As the great theorist Max Weber argued, bureaucracies are rooted in norms of impersonality.[18] Unlike the kindly country doctors of yesteryear whose work involved home visits and the involvement of the whole family, contemporary healers are bound by bureaucratic rules, legal obligations to maintain confidentiality, a mountain of paperwork associated with insurance payments, and HMO regulations detailing who can be treated for what and for how long.[19] These contextual dimensions of professional work, combined with the training of doctors whose expertise is increasingly restricted to particular body parts, ensures a bureaucratic system that grows ever more remote from the humane treatment of human problems.

I suspect that the distress and anger felt toward doctors are magnified in the case of psychiatry. It is, after all, the area of medicine considered the least "scientific," in which the expertise of practitioners is potentially most questionable. Although fads and fashions come and go with regularity in all areas of medicine, the transformations in the field of psychiatry have been dramatic over the last fifty years.[20] Today, conventional talk therapy and psychoanalysis, so long the staples of training in psychiatry, are either marginalized during medical training or eradicated completely from the curriculum. The prevailing ideology of American psychiatry is that mental illnesses are brain diseases to be treated pharmacologically. Claims of tremendous advancement in psychiatric medicine routinely appear in the public media. However, for the families gripped by someone's mental illness, the media hype is rarely matched by effective treatments. Thus, not only do caregivers and patients feel diminished by bureaucratic processes, they eventually grow dubious about psychiatrists' claims to expertise. The combination of shabby treatment, high initial expectations, and poor results is certainly a prescription for cynicism.

> I don't have a stereotype against therapy or anything like that. [Well], maybe I did have some sort of . . . reservations about going to see someone. I mean, I had no respect for the woman, the psychiatrist, who dealt with my mom. [Now] I don't trust any type of psychotropic medication. . . . I saw firsthand all of the different side effects and things it would do to her. Sometimes her teeth would chatter. She would have tremor type things and it was totally scary seeing your mom going through something like that. I mean, I just saw how messed up she was and I couldn't help but think that at least a small part of it was just the drugs. I am sure some people really do need medication. I think that a lot of times doctors, and by that I mean psychiatrists, like go for a quick fix and so they don't really monitor their patients and [see] what is really going on. . . . I think that definitely this doctor kind of . . . gave up on my mom. Her way of dealing with it was like, "Okay, we'll just give you a different medicine."
>
> RESEARCH ASSISTANT, *age twenty-three, daughter*

⤶

> I think they [doctors] process them, basically. They process her. They get frustrated because they can't do anything, and they say, "Sorry." You know? "She's not committable. Good luck. Have a nice day." And they walk away, because they can do that. I think there are a few people that have been pretty good. They've gone a little bit of an extra mile. I don't know what to expect from them either. You know, it's a job for them. I mean, you know, how much are they supposed to take on? I don't know. . . . She's seeing some doctor

now, and I'm not really too happy with him, because I think he would basically take the fees, give her four medications when she only needs one—I pay for all that—and go, "Well, see you next week."

ACCOUNTANT, age thirty-five, daughter

⌒

Yeah, I am pretty cynical and that is because I haven't seen much help. I am not cynical about the people who are trying to treat them. I mean, I know that there are good, caring people who really have their hearts in the right places and they really want to help my mother and my brother and even myself, when I suffered from depression. But I am cynical about the narrow focus of the mental health industry world. Yeah, I am cynical about the emphasis on medication. I am cynical about the ignorance that I feel the mental health world has regarding sort of completely changing their angle, I guess you could say. It seems to me that the [drug] model isn't working too well. People who are suffering from schizophrenia. . . . they say with certain medications, the new medications, a person can lead an almost normal life. I feel like you are really insulting somebody's spirit, when you tell them that they can lead an almost normal life.

ARTIST, age thirty-three, son and brother

The perspectives you are hearing here from caregivers are created, in large measure, by the frustration that inevitably accompanies their efforts to find effective treatment. Their anger at doctors may be justified in particular instances, but we need to remember that those who work in and for the system, who are part of the system, are also themselves, in varying degrees, controlled by the system. The last respondent likely had it right when he said "I am not cynical about the people who are trying to treat them. I mean, I know that there are good, caring people who really have their hearts in the right places and they really want to help." If we could interview doctors, nurses, social workers, and various hospital staff, we would no doubt find them equally frustrated by the limitations imposed by HMOs, bureaucratic regulations, insurance companies, the absence of outpatient facilities, the lack of parity accorded physical and mental illnesses, the limitations of their own knowledge, and a legal structure that sometimes blocks the treatment of catastrophically ill people. Like those they serve, professionals are also subject to the vagaries, impersonality, paradoxes, and inconsistencies that characterize any large system of interconnected bureaucracies.

For caregivers, a family member's tribulations with mental illness require that they unwillingly embark on a crash course, without much guidance, in how to negotiate different parts of a complicated system. Thus far, you have heard about the difficulties surrounding their encounters with police, crisis teams, hospitals, and mental health professionals, particularly doctors. In the following section, this chapter comes full circle since I began by describing one mother's plea via an open letter for someone, anyone, to help her get medical insurance for her daughter. Unless they are independently wealthy, caregivers must find a way to pay for a family member's treatment. Difficulties with police, crisis teams, getting an ill person hospitalized, or extracting information from psychiatric experts sometimes seemed modest compared to the problems of obtaining "benefits."

Paying for Care

I am an intelligent enough person to follow most complex discussions. Still, like Carol, whose words and concerns open this chapter, I remain baffled by how the mental health system works, but especially confounded by the bureaucratic gymnastics required to find proper insurance or government benefits to cover the medical costs of mental illness. Over and over in the MDDA group, the conversation turns to the cost of health care and the impenetrability of the process for getting benefits. No matter how many times I hear conversation about the difficulties of qualifying for social security payments (SSI), social security disability payments (SSDI), private insurance plans, MassHealth (the Massachusetts State Health Insurance System), and the complex relationships among these plans, my eyes glaze over.

Every now and then, there is a guest speaker at MDDA who is invited to address the group because he or she is an "expert" on the system. In fact, one of the clearest presentations was made by a woman who now earns her livelihood by successfully securing government disability insurance for her clients. Her expertise, attained over many years, involves knowing just how to negotiate the system, how to fill out forms, how to reach the "right" person, how to "stay on the case" with the appropriate bureaucrats, how to cope with eligibility requirements that seem to change nearly daily, and how to change the application after the nearly automatic first denial (a denial that the unschooled often take at face value). Even after her relatively clear explanation, I still felt perplexed.

One thing seems clear. It is that however good their puzzle-solving skills, those who have not routinely dealt with the insurance system for years find it mystifying. Nearly always, the job of applying for various benefits falls to healthy family members. How could it be otherwise? If people with relatively clear heads cannot fathom an always changing bureaucratic system, how possibly could a mentally ill person without family resources ever obtain benefits? I want you to hear how some of the people I interviewed described their frustration in figuring out finances. Normally, when I have people speak in this book, my choice is based on three criteria. First, I want you to hear from people whose perspectives and experiences are representative. Second, I want to give lots of people a chance to speak. Third, all other things being equal, I am more likely to quote someone who is articulate and coherent. If, however, you have some trouble following the comments below, it is because the speaker is genuinely confused. Read on to experience a bit of that confusion.

> Yeah, my attitude is, that given the resources or lack thereof of the family, that my sister should have applied for benefits earlier, gone to some place that would retroactively accept the DMH [Department

of Mental Health] benefits. Look at the quality of that care and if
that wasn't getting anywhere, investigate the next step. That's what
I would have done. If this doesn't work, there is no place to go but
up, and who is going to pay for the next round? . . . People are going
to be expecting that after three months she is going to work full-
time? I mean what is . . . that is what I really don't. . . . Well this
particular program won't take, you know . . . it's a private [program].
You have to just pay for it and she doesn't have an expensive insurance policy that would cover it and I guess for her to be determined
for Department of Mental Health eligibility she had to agree to sign
some paperwork and she didn't until very very late in the process.
I think . . . you know . . . I don't even know if her disability has
kicked in yet. About a month before that she applied for disability
and then nobody told us "Well, there is a separate set of paper work
for Department of Mental Health status for the state hospital benefits
than there is for just receiving a monthly check from Social
Security."

TECHNOLOGY LICENSER, *age thirty three, sister*

Others described the arduous efforts required to become eligible
for benefits:

[I spent] hours and hours and hours on the phone. I had to find
out how to get him health benefits from the beginning. I can't even
tell you how many hours I spent. He has no idea what I've done to
find this and that and all this stuff.

DAY-CARE ATTENDANT, *age fifty-five, spouse*

↩

We got him onto Mass Health on our own by filling out, seriously,
thirty pages of paperwork. I remember he is laying in bed totally
depressed and I'm asking him questions and filling it out for him.
And some of the questions are just so funny. You know, "Did you
ever work at a job where you lifted over fifty pounds?" Just silly
things like that. I remember not filling some of that out because I

thought, "This is so ridiculous. What does this have to do [with anything]? . . . It took us three days to fill out the paperwork if that tells you anything. . . . Now, he is also on disability which we did by going through [names consultant]. They got him on disability. Thank God because those papers . . . that was probably fifty pages.

GRADUATE STUDENT, *age twenty-eight, wife*

↜

My fear, as a parent, is what happens if I'm not here. Well, I've talked to her brother because of the insurance and financial responsibilities and things like that. If she gets anything from a trust, she doesn't have any insurance. Her last hospitalization was $62,000. And, she had her insurance pay for the first month. Fortunately, I had been talking with the SSI office, and had done all of these things that the hospital should have been doing, [but] that they didn't do. Like arranging [things] and knowing her insurance was going to expire. All the paperwork should have been in place for her SSI. I mean, when she's in the hospital, I can't tell you how many hours a day I spent on the phone talking to these people about all these different issues and what is available and things like that. But the hospital did call her and say that she had an outstanding balance of $62,000. And, this is what the hospital does to someone who just got out of the psychiatric hospital. [When] half of her problem is stress that has caused her to go over the edge.

RETIRED SECRETARY, *age fifty-eight, mother*

As with so many other aspects of caring for the mentally ill, the very character of the illness compromises efforts to qualify for benefits. You will remember from earlier discussions that mentally ill people frequently deny their problem. Sometimes financially strapped family members cannot even begin the process of securing Social Security disability insurance because their ill parent, spouse, sibling, or child refuses to acknowledge that they are disabled by mental illness. Even among those who clearly perceive that they have a mental illness, there is often a reluctance to admit that they are sufficiently ill to fall into the class of the "disabled." Ill people often recoil at the word "disability." The emotions surrounding disability insurance go well beyond the paperwork involved in the process. Rather, and far more important, to apply for and obtain disability payments involves an unwelcome transformation of identity. To receive the insurance is a kind of affirmation that one is, indeed, "mentally ill." It is a label many are unwilling to accept.

> This is so frustrating. She won't agree that she is mentally ill, so she won't you know [apply for benefits]. She wouldn't get any benefits, so we were basically supporting her. She had no money, so it was like, you know, trying to buy her groceries. The house is falling apart, but where are your priorities? Trying to keep the bills going and I was struggling, we were all struggling. It's awful. I mean we didn't want this to happen, but she had a major heart attack. So . . . the good in that was that she was able to qualify for a disability and she would agree to *that* disability. So now she has a disability income, not much.
>
> ACCOUNTANT, *age thirty-five, daughter*

↩

> My sister has absolutely no medical insurance and has only agreed three weeks ago to apply for Medicare/Medicaid Department of Mental Health status, all that kind of thing. . . . I mean, we forced [*names hospital*] to figure it out. . . . It came out [in conversation] that my sister had been told what paperwork needed to be filled out and she refused to fill it out. So that was what really held up the process, that my sister just didn't want to be termed a mental patient. She just never wanted to fill out paperwork to get these benefits.
>
> TECHNOLOGY LICENSER, *age thirty-three, sister*

I have repeatedly maintained that mental illness is highly contagious. As multiple social science studies show, the unremitting stress associated with caregiving makes people sick.[21] Easily a majority of the sixty folks I interviewed require the help of therapists in order to survive the ordeal of a loved one's mental illness. Many are themselves being treated for severe depression. By this point in my description, you should understand the variety of stresses that define the plight of caregivers. Certainly one of the most powerful stresses affecting the health of caregivers arises from the financial uncertainty that accompanies the onset of mental illness. Unless they are fortunate enough to have substantial private insurance, they must live with the constant and frightening question, "How will we pay?" I imagine that the sort of constant money anxiety felt by many of my respondents corresponds to the paralyzing fear felt by millions of Americans without adequate health insurance or, worse, no insurance at all.

> Oh God, I wish we were the Kennedys. You know, we're upper-middle class, I guess, but we can't afford [the kind of care he needs]. Even if he had private insurance, it would have run out by now. There's a place called [names private hospital]. Have you ever heard of that? It's a place where the wealthy can send their mentally ill relatives. We can't afford that. And, you know, we have a decent income, but we can't afford that. So, I don't know what the answer is. He's on Medicaid . . . and stuck in the public mental health system.
>
> SECRETARY, *age fifty-one, mother*

↜

> I don't know [what we will do]. I don't know. A friend of mine who is a psychiatric nurse . . . said that if worse came to worse, I guess there is emergency Medicare or Medicaid they could get him on right away, but that is not going to help a lot with the medications in-between [hospitalizations]. All the medications are so expensive. . . . My exasperation is who is going to pay for it now? I am not going to lie. I am deeply in debt for having tried to help him get on his feet. I thought he was going to get on his feet and it hasn't happened.
>
> HOME HEALTH AIDE, *age forty-four, mother*

〜

I don't know how they (parents) are going to retire and I'm worried
sick about that. I am so worried about that. He is on Social Security.
She earns money. But if he suddenly needs inpatient mental health
care, his insurance doesn't cover it. They are up a creek.

LAWYER, *age thirty-three, daughter*

〜

We have major medical—Blue Cross/Blue Shield—but our co-
payments are choking us. Our co-payments are probably as high as
the insurance. Every time you have a doctor's visit . . . it's ten or
twenty dollars. The insurance pays for medication, but you have a
co-payment. So, you're talking hundreds of dollars a week. It's just
pissing away the money on all this stuff.

ART RESTORER, *age fifty, father*

The broadest, most enduring theoretical task of sociology is to
understand how human behavior is simultaneously shaped by the
day-to-day, face-to-face encounters we have with others and the
larger social structures within which these daily interactions take
place. The "paradox of culture," as some describe it, is that humans
are a social product and that culture is a human product.[22] Culture
begins to create us from the moment we are wrapped in either the
pink or blue blanket. However, once created, the human capacity
to reflect, think, interpret, and imagine lets us refashion the culture
that made us. Social life, then, is an ongoing dialectical process
between the power we have to shape our own lives and the reality
that the dramas of daily life occur within larger historical and institutional settings over which we often have little control.

As a social psychologist, I believe that any attempt to understand
the operation of society that neglects the processes governing social
interaction will be theoretically dissatisfying. Ultimately a society is
composed of persons interacting with one another. All explanations
of human behavior must in some way account for individuals' in-

tentions, motives, and subjective understandings of the situation in which they act. Accordingly, my focus throughout the first five chapters was on the "micro worlds" of caregivers' immediate experiences with an ill family member. I detailed how those interactions continuously shape caregivers' perceptions of their obligations to an ill family member. In this chapter, my attention turned to those larger, more abstract, and remote social structures composing the mental health system. You have seen how efforts to deal with and make sense of "the system" profoundly influence how family members experience their caregiving.

These days, there is quite a lot of talk about how our health care system is failing us. Astounding numbers of Americans are without health insurance.[23] What becomes of people with catastrophic illness surely reflects America's class structure and the gross inequities in resources that characterize it. A failing health system can mean life or death for people. The accounts in this chapter suggest that the mental health system is badly broken. Story after story confirms the view of the woman who said, "The system is just so ridiculous. . . . Despite wonderful people being in the system, [it's] so flawed and it's going to cost lives." Another person agreed by saying, "It's gotta be fixed. It's so messed up. They haven't cared about the mentally ill because the mentally ill can't fight for themselves. They are dismissed. We need to get together and advocate for our loved ones because no one else is doing it."

Forty years ago, the conditions in America's mental hospitals were intolerable and a shameful measure of our ignorance about and disregard for the mentally ill. Today, things are better. Scientific advances have been made that warrant a measure of optimism about the prospects for the estimated twenty million mentally ill people in the United States. An escalating number of newspaper stories, television programs, and books about their plight suggests that the situation of the mentally ill might be slowly emerging from the shadows of our national consciousness. Clearly, though, we have a long way to go. The mentally ill are still feared, stigmatized, and largely ignored. We have a double health standard—one attitude toward the physically ill and quite another toward the mentally ill. In both cases, however, policies directed toward providing quality health care for everyone in America lag far behind the pleading voices of the family members who know firsthand how badly the system is failing them and their loved ones.

If we want to understand why we lack the national will to fix our ailing health system, we need to consider our cultural attitudes about care itself. I have been arguing throughout this book that boundaries of obligation between healthy and ill family members are constructed in the flow of daily life. At the same time, what we feel and how we act toward an ill relative cannot be understood apart from cultural mandates about the meanings attached to care. In the next chapter, I want to continue the "macro" or "structural" level of analysis I have initiated here. To understand both our national policies toward the mentally ill and much of the confusion voiced by caregivers throughout this book, we need to examine the cultural roots of our disposition to care or not to care. With the help of those who have written on the matter, the last chapter examines the extraordinary cultural ambivalence about caring that characterizes America society.

SEVEN

Caring in Postmodern America

*If I am not for myself, who will be for me? If I am not
for others, what am I?*

RABBI HILLEL

Among our commitments that seem least negotiable are those to
our immediate family. Presumably, moral persons will look after
kin *no matter what*. However, this expectation rubs against the
equally powerful cultural idea that we should be free to fulfill our
personal desires. Wally Lamb's recent novel, *I Know This Much Is
True*, centers on the lifelong connections between two identical twin
brothers, one of whom succumbs to schizophrenia in his late teens.[1]
Much of the novel is about the binding commitment between Dominick and his sick brother, Thomas. The tension throughout the
book is between caring and freedom, between fulfilling a commitment to a brother and realizing one's own aspirations. With an
artist's rendering, Lamb gets at the complicated, opposed, and profoundly distressing feelings that arise when caregivers cannot resolve
the conflict between the moral mandates to care for a family member and personal freedom. Here is how Dominick describes his
feelings during a meeting with a therapist:

> "You want to know what it's like for me? *Do* you? It's like ... it's
> like ... my brother has been an anchor on me my whole life. Pulling me down. Even *before* he got sick. ... An anchor. ... And you
> know what I get? I get just enough rope to break the surface. To

breathe. But I am never, ever going to . . . You know what I used to think? I used to think that eventually—you know, sooner or later— I was going to get away from him. Cut the chord, you know? But here I am, forty years old and I'm still down at the nuthouse, running interference for my fucking. . . . Treading water. It's like . . . like. . . . And I *hate* him sometimes. I do. I'll admit it. I really hate him. But you know something? Here's the *really* fucked-up part. Nobody *else* better say anything—nobody else better even look at him cross-eyed or I'll. . . . And the thing is, I think I finally *get* it, you know?"

"Get what, Dominick?"

"That he's my *curse*. My *anchor*. That I'm just going to tread water for the rest of my whole life. That he *is* my whole life! My fucking, fucked-up brother. I'm just going to tread water, just breathe . . . and that's it. I'm never going to get away from him! Never!"

"The other day? Last week, it was? I went to the convenience store. My girlfriend says, 'We're out of milk, Dominick. Go get some milk.' So I go to the convenience store and I put a gallon of milk on the counter and this clerk—this fat fuck with orange hair and a pierced nose—he's just. . . . He was *staring* at me like . . . like I'm . . ."

"Like you were what?"

"Like I'm *him!* *Thomas*. Which I . . . Which I probably will be before I'm through. I mean, we're twins, right? It's going to happen eventually, isn't it?"

"What, exactly, do you think is going to happen Dominick?"

"He's going to pull me under. I'm going to drown."[2]

Like the people who have spoken in earlier chapters, Dominick is pushed and pulled by strongly opposing forces. His psychic life, his internal torment, reflects extraordinary ambivalence. The dictionary defines ambivalence as "uncertainty or fluctuation, especially when caused by inability to make a choice or a simultaneous desire to say or do two opposite things." A second definition, designated as psychological, describes ambivalence as "the coexistence within an individual of positive and negative feelings toward the same person, object, or action, simultaneously drawing him in opposite directions."

The editors of Webster's dictionary are correct in identifying ambivalence as a psychological condition insofar as it is individuals who feel the ambivalence and experience it as their own internal struggle. What the dictionary definition does not acknowledge is that the terms of the ambivalence—the simultaneity of opposite feelings—stem ultimately from society. People are ambivalent because culture dictates expectations that potentially conflict with one another. Dominick's ambivalence toward his brother arises from two powerful and apparently contradictory cultural messages. One is that we are to love, protect, and care for family members regardless of the personal cost. The second is that we have the right—indeed, we have the obligation—to pursue personal happiness. After all, we "only go around once!" Dominick's internal pain, like that expressed by the caregivers in this book, arises from the dual and paradoxical expectations that we be obligated both to self and to others.

The respondents in this study nearly unanimously say that the hardest thing about dealing with a mentally ill family member is never knowing whether their caregiving choices are correct. Time and again, family members raise questions about closeness and distance, independence and dependence, giving one's self to others fully or preserving themselves by disengaging. Line drawing is part of every discussion about coping because of the inevitable feeling that wherever they have drawn the line it is the "wrong" place. To give money or to withhold it? To allow a child to live at home or demand that they live independently? To accept a spouse's failure to work as a product of their illness or insist that they exercise greater personal responsibility? To rescue a family member in trouble or let them struggle with the consequences of their actions? These are the kinds of questions that cause caregiving agony.

Drawing inspiration from the global perspectives of writers like

Thomas Hobbes, Jean Jacques Rousseau, John Locke, Sigmund Freud, John Rawls, Adam Smith, and Talcott Parsons, contemporary theorists arrive at fundamentally different conclusions about the origin and operation of social obligations. While I acknowledge the importance of this conversation and the aesthetically pleasing character of some of the theories proposed, something vitally important is missing. The theories begin and end with abstract principles, propositions, and axioms. In all of this, the implicit assumption is that, whichever propositions are correct, human beings make their moral choices unreflectively because they are simply guided by abstract principles. After a wonderfully detailed treatment of these ideas, Alan Wolfe comes to the conclusion that "what [we] need is an approach that, instead of insisting that it has all the right answers, tries to locate a sense of moral obligation in common sense, ordinary emotions, and everyday life."[3]

This book has, in fact, been directed at trying to understand the kind of "local interpretations" that caregivers must make of their immediate circumstances; my data speak to the "micro worlds" of everyday life. You have seen that the people I interviewed cannot assess their obligations apart from the particular contingencies they face at home. At the same time, it would be a mistake to believe that their assessments and interpretations are somehow independent from the ways that the broader culture dictates the character of obligations to sick persons. The purpose of this chapter is to raise the level of the analysis beyond the day-to-day, nitty-gritty requirements of caring and look at the range of rhetoric that surrounds our ideas about the moral thing to do when a family member is incapacitated. Beyond that, my aim is to show how cultural ideas influence a society's concrete choices about the resources it will provide for its less fortunate members.

Because there is the potential for the idea to get lost in the pages to follow, I want to once again emphasize that mental illness, *by its very nature*, physically and emotionally exhausts family caregivers. Just a few days before writing these words I listened to a husband and wife plaintively ask others in the Family and Friends group whether their torment would ever end. No one even tried to respond to this semi-rhetorical question. Still, knowing that those hearing the question at least understood it properly, gave relief. There is, I'm suggesting, a universal dimension to caregivers' pain brought about by mental illness. And so, even though I believe there are cultural differences in the way people experience pain and suffering, such an observation does not diminish the essential truth that mental illness is horrible for anyone touched by it, wherever and whenever it occurs. Having said this, I want to argue that it would, nevertheless, be incomplete to understand the interpretive problems of caregivers *only* in terms of a terribly confounding illness.

A very fundamental *cultural* question surrounds the interpretive difficulties documented in earlier pages. It is a global question about what we owe to ourselves, what we owe to others, and what we think society owes us. It is a question about what it means to be a moral and caring person at the turn of the twentieth century in the United States. To understand fully the confusion respondents have been expressing throughout this volume, we need to look at the paradoxes and complexities surrounding issues of obligation to self and to others in American society. Every time family caregivers speak in this volume their comments reflect cultural values. Each expression of the "right" or "wrong" thing to do arises from one or another cultural script.

Of course, the idea of culture has a long and rich tradition in the social sciences. Culture is generally conceived to be a kind of blueprint for living, a set of beliefs, ideas, and sentiments that guide our lives socially and morally. In small, simple societies cultural requirements are typically uniform and provide guidelines for a proper life shared by all the members of that culture. On the positive side, such homogenous cultures protect people, embrace them, so to speak, by giving clear meaning to their daily lives, and ultimately, therefore, by providing the basis for social regularity, predictability, and order. On the negative side, however, homogeneous cultures can be stifling as they leave little room for divergent

thinking and the inevitable human impulses that chafe against socially constructed beliefs and expectations.[4] However, as Kai Erikson
shows, even in relatively homogeneous societies, "Life is frequently
a thing of ambivalence and tension, of contradiction and conflict;
and these are exactly the elements one hears the least about in most
social science descriptions of culture."[5]

Erikson analyzed how a small Appalachian mining community
responded to a humanly produced disaster—a dam that burst, producing a wall of water that destroyed everything its path and killed
125 people. Like all cultures, in greater or lesser degree, Appalachian
culture is bounded by motifs that seem contradictory. Mountain
life, his study revealed, is characterized by a sharp tension between
the miners' love of tradition and an ethic of personal freedom, by
a deep contrast between self-assertion and resignation, by a simultaneous self-centeredness and group-centeredness, between feelings
of ability and disability, between a sense of independence and a
need for dependence. Similar contradictions, tensions, paradoxes,
or ambivalence are part of every culture, although they generally
become more overt and acute as societies become increasingly complex, modern, and diverse in composition.

In the case of the miners, cultural paradoxes did not become
apparent until the disaster utterly disrupted everyday life in their
community. Only then could the taken-for-granted culture, with all
its internal contradictions, became manifestly problematic. Analogously, mental illness invariably constitutes a family catastrophe and
thus reveals cultural tensions that, in the absence of tragedy, are
much easier to live with and resolve. Americans, I shall argue, are
deeply conflicted about what they owe themselves and what they
owe others. Our culture, far more than most, provides mixed messages and viewpoints about this central life issue. No single script
or blueprint guides our judgments about proper feelings, thoughts,
behaviors, and relationships. We listen to a pluralism of cultural
voices dictating conflicting messages. It is a cacophony of moral
relativism that some say defines the condition of postmodern
America.[6]

Postmodernity and Individuality

All of social life involves a tension between freedom and constraint. Living in a society inevitably involves a trade-off between personal liberty and commitment to others. We judge some societies as immoral because they allow virtually no personal freedoms and others because they seem unable to constrain their members. For much of its history, American democracy provided a healthy balance between commitment and freedom. For a long time, the pursuit of personal happiness and individual goals seemed compatible with a set of cultural values that Americans willingly embraced and held them together as a nation. Now a group of sociologists who call themselves communitarians argue that the balance between freedom and constraint, between rights and responsibilities has fallen dangerously out of whack.[7]

I should say that the founders of my discipline worried about just such an eventuality. Sociology was borne in the throes of the industrial revolution that enveloped mid-nineteenth-century Europe. Although their conceptual visions differed in important respects, classical sociological theorists were united in their view that people's connections to each other and to society itself were increasingly loosened as societies modernized. Another way to say this is that nineteenth-century theorists worried about the coherence of culture. They worried that the fabric of culture was fraying under the influence of "modernism." Whereas culture once provided clear guidelines for nearly all aspects of life in agrarian communities, the urban world was far more fragmented. The result, writers like Emile Durkheim, Karl Marx, and Max Weber argued, was a decreased integration of persons into societies.

At the heart of their worries was the tension between individualism and communalism. The German theorist Ferdinand Tönnies distinguished what he termed *Gemeinschaft* and *Gesellschaft*.[8] Gemeinschaft, literally translated as community, described the tight bonds of people living in agrarian societies. In contrast, Gesellschaft, translated as "society," referred to the impersonal, highly segmented social organization of urban places. In contrast to the impersonality of industrial cities, members of small communities related to each other as kin. They were bound together by a tight, coherent, and mutually held set of cultural rules that defined proper behaviors in all areas of social life. Comparing his two types, Tönnies wrote that "Gesellschaft . . . superficially resembles the Gemeinschaft in so far as the individuals live and dwell together peacefully. However, in the Gemeinschaft they remain essentially united in spite of separating factors, whereas in the Gesellschaft they are essentially separated in spite of all uniting factors."[9]

Nineteenth-century thinkers tended to romanticize the sort of Gemeinschaft-like relations described by Tönnies. Although culture certainly integrated people in simpler societies, there was a huge price to pay—the blunting of individualism. On the whole, though, nineteenth-century theorists feared the suffocating potential of communities less than the atomizing and individualizing effects of the emerging industrial world. They were unanimous in their view that people were less morally constrained in modern societies because their commitments to communities of all sorts had become far more tenuous.

Although sociologists have always claimed the importance of community to a healthy society, it is only in the last decade or so that communitarians have been actively calling for a revitalization of community. One of the gurus of the communitarian movement, Amitai Etzioni, refers to the need for a basic reorientation of cultural values when he says, "What America needs, above all, is a change in the way we approach things, what we value and what we devalue, a change of heart."[10] Communitarians have been warning us about the erosion of fundamental American values and the deterioration of private and public morality. The deterioration, they say, is reflected in the weakening of such essential institutions as the family and the school. Moreover, the decline of these institutions and the corresponding increases in crime and corruption are presumably the product of a society that has created a lopsided and dangerous imbalance of "rights" over "responsibilities."

As communitarians read American history, traditional morality has been in a particularly sharp tailspin over the last few decades. Although the "happy days" of the fifties also disenfranchised women and maintained sharp racial divisions, Americans still emphasized an ethic of personal responsibility during those years. Certainly the turmoil of the 1960s and 1970s began to significantly reshape the society as young people questioned virtually all significant American values and the institutions that produced them. The demand for greater "participatory democracy" during those years, Etzioni maintains, went too far and drifted into "rampant moral confusion and social anarchy."[11]

By the 1980s Americans had become deeply imbued with the idea that the society owed them all kinds of "rights" without any corresponding responsibilities. Etzioni shares a piece of data that crystallized for him the kind of damaging imbalance that had been created between rights and responsibilities. It was a finding that the majority of young people in America believed that they had the right to a jury trial while indicating at the same time that they would not want to serve on a jury![12] Indeed, by the Reagan years of the 1980s, Gordon Gekko, the protagonist in the movie *Wall Street* could passionately claim that "greed is good" for America. The country had clearly moved from a "we" to a "me" orientation to such a degree that the historian Christopher Lasch could describe America as a "culture of narcissism."[13] Etzioni comments on these transformations and the ethic of his communitarian philosophy.

> The eighties tried to turn vice into virtue by elevating the unbridled pursuit of self-interest and greed to the level of a social virtue. It turned out that the *economy* could thrive (at least for a while) if people watched out only for themselves.... But it has become evident that a *society* cannot function well given such self-centered, me-istic orientations. It requires a set of do's and don'ts, a set of moral values, that guides people toward what is decent and encourages them to avoid that which is not.[14]

Other contemporary theorists sustain the same view, emphasizing the degree to which an ethic of "expressive individualism" minimizes persons' felt obligation to each other. Robert Bellah writes that "individualism lies at the very core of American culture. ... We believe in the dignity, indeed the sacredness, of the individual."[15] Postmodern writers say that contemporary American society is defined by increasingly short-lived and superficial relationships, geographical mobility that diminishes our commitment to place, and a mass media that confronts us with multiple and contradictory points of view on nearly everything.[16] Zygmunt Bauman has described the "postmodern self" as composed of "momentary identities, identities 'for today', until further notice identities."[17] Such momentary and fluid identities, which are furthermore dedicated to self-enhancement, conspire to minimize our sense of responsibility to each other. Thus, the prevailing opinion of sociologists from the nineteenth century to the present seems to be that we may live in a world *with* others, but an ethic of individualism makes it increasingly difficult to live *for* others.

The kind of individualism decried by Etzioni and others is surely reflected in the cultural values underlying a number of sectors of the society. In the world of work, for example, at least for "white collar" workers, there has been, until recently, a kind of *quid pro quo*. Organizations provided long-term security and received, in turn, worker loyalty, commitment, and responsibility. Loyalty, responsibility, security, commitment. These are the binding features of social systems, the glue that sustains the bond between individuals and social institutions. Unhappily, America's emerging "postindustrial" economy seems to have fundamentally altered the meaning of work for many by eroding loyalty, commitment, and mutual responsibility between organizations and workers.[18] Critics of capitalism, however, would maintain that the negative effects of capitalism on human relationships are far more inclusive than those in the workplace. In a more general way, the values underpinning capitalism are evident in a large variety of face-to-face encounters.

Competition, for example, is one of the cornerstones of capitalism. Advocates of capitalism maintain that competition is a necessary ingredient in both maintaining organizational efficiency and motivating individuals. On the negative side, however, competition pits individuals against each other, diminishes trust, and generally dehumanizes relationships. Capitalism contributes to a culture of inauthenticity. In a society in which everything and everyone is evaluated by their profit potential, individuals are aware that they are constantly being manipulated, seduced, and conned by those who want to sell them or "take them." In a world held together by appearances and a tissue of illusions and deceptions, everyone becomes an enemy of sorts whose motives cannot be accepted at face value. In short, the abstract values of capitalism "trickle down" to everyday consciousness in a way that induces human beings to distrust and withdraw from each other. In contemporary America, characterized by a kind of hyperindividuality, the "choice" to care becomes problematic in a way that would have been unfathomable in simpler societies. Patricia Benner and Suzanne Gordon write that

> Caring thus becomes a free choice made by human beings who are depicted as rational choicemakers. These rational choicemakers can stand back and objectively choose whether or not to care for friends, loved ones, colleagues, or strangers. They are said to care because they "feel like it," and "get something out of it," just as they choose not to care if it "feels" inconvenient or doesn't feel good. This instrumental frame not only turns caring into a choice, it also transforms connectedness, responsiveness, and interdependence into signs of moral lapse or sources of embarrassment or shame.[19]

Postmodernity and Communality

Although writers are correct to emphasize America's ethic of individualism, it would be wrong to think that cultural ideas about community and strict mandates about obligation to others have disappeared. A more accurate description is that Americans believe in community and individualism *at the same time*. We are provided scripts or narratives that stress both. The postmodern paradox is that we are expected to be committed both to ourselves and to others at the same time. This paradox is evident in a wide range of cultural stories, some of which celebrate connection and community and others that applaud individualism. It is no wonder that caregivers are confused about boundary lines. They are taught to believe simultaneously in the sanctity of the self and of attachments to others. The underlying tension of postmodernity is the urge of persons to be involved and uninvolved, connected and disconnected at the same time.

The coexisting tensions between versions of individualism and commitment to others is nicely illustrated in Robert Wuthnow's book *Acts of Compassion*.[20] Although there are sharp differences between the requirements of full-time caring for desperately sick family members and the feelings of compassion that lead people to volunteer their time in soup kitchens and the like, Wuthnow's analysis turns on the coexistence of seemingly opposed cultural values. Data from surveys and personal interviews indicate that Americans are deeply involved in a range of charitable efforts. They give huge amounts of time and money to this "third sector" of the economy.[21] Moreover, his interviews indicate that large numbers of Americans express in word and deed a fundamental altruism that seems at odds with images of the United States as a place where people are interested *only* in their personal welfare. At the end of his first chapter, Wuthnow sets out an important research question. He asks, "How is it that we as a people are able to devote billions of hours to volunteer activities, to show care and compassion in so many ways to those around us, and still be a nation of individualists who pride ourselves on personal freedom, individual success, and the pursuit of self-interest?"[22] His answer is that we incorporate both sets of values into our thinking. It's not one or the other.

Other analyses point to countervailing cultural forces that blunt radical individualism, emphasizing as they do our connection to each other. For example, in her book *Misery and Company: Sympathy in Everyday Life* Candace Clark describes, documents, and analyzes the deep cultural roots of compassion and sympathy.[23]

Clark's book catalogues the cultural rules that surround the expression and the acceptance of sympathy. She persuasively maintains that sympathy is an integral part of the glue that holds a culture together. Clark shows that sympathy rules are well elaborated and clearly understood in the United States. Properly socialized persons know when and how much sympathy to extend in a wide array of circumstances. Sympathy is to be extended to persons, who through no fault of their own, face "bad luck" situations. In the wide array of such circumstances we know that the expression of too much or too little sympathy will mark us as deviant. Moreover, she argues that there are "sympathy entrepreneurs" who are constantly engaged in an enterprise to expand the circumstances for which sympathy is rightly expressed. The Hallmark card company, for example, has a significant investment in shaping the cultural norms surrounding the expression of sympathy.

Clark's work testifies to the fact that while we elevate the self, we also expect moral persons to maintain certain commitments. Even as postmodernity fosters the ascendancy of the self, we retain strong cultural convictions that we owe others sympathy, commitment, and caring. This is not to say that individuals are disingenuous when they feel compassion for another, when their heart goes out to them. That their feelings of compassion are socially profiled does not make them any less real. The social origin of all feelings does not diminish their reality because, as Russell Jacoby puts it, "the social does not [simply] 'influence' the private, it dwells within it."[24] Even those feelings that we think arise from the deepest preserves of our individual hearts and souls arise from society. Of all such feelings that might engage our attention here, love deserves special mention. Americans' conception of romantic love demonstrates our simultaneous yearnings for connection and separation.

The advice columns of daily newspapers, television programming, and popular fiction all indicate the extent to which the depth and quality of our intimate ties occupy our time and thoughts. Even in the context of the sort of individualism that pushes us away from each other, our attitudes about love reveal how much we want to care for others and to be cared about. We all expect to "fall" in love and from early adolescence on we wait for that moment when "that old black magic has us in its spell." The "romantic ideal" is celebrated in music, art, cinema, and literature.[25] One particularly thriving industry capitalizes on our love of love, our need for intimacy, and our wish for total, timeless commitment. Although romance novels do not appear on the *New York Times* bestseller lists, their sales easily match those of other bestsellers. In 1988, Harlequin books, one of the largest publishers of romance novels, sold 202 million books, a rate of 550,000 per day.[26] Perhaps, though, such sales figures are evidence that we rarely find the intimacy we seek, that, as another popular song put it a while back, millions of people are desperately "looking for love in all the wrong places."

It may not be an exaggeration to say that love has become a social problem of sorts in America. The difficulties in establishing the connections we dearly wish for are affirmed by a trip to any local bookstore. The shelves in the psychology and "self-help" sections are routinely filled with titles promising formulas for the right ways and places to find love. Thomas McNight's and Robert Phillips's *Love Tactics* provides "effective techniques for winning over or getting back the one you love." Susan Page promises to answer the question *If I'm So Wonderful Why Am I Still Single?"* Straight to the point of this chapter, Jordan and Margaret Paul's book speaks about the quintessentially American danger that, in finding love, we might lose ourselves. Their book is entitled *Do I Have to Give Up Me to be Loved by You?* Apparently, the problem of finding and maintaining love is greater for women than for men. On the same shelves you can find Susan Kelly's *Why Men Stray, Why Men Stay.* There are, however, no comparable books explaining to men how to recognize a "commitment-phobic" woman before she breaks your heart.

The cultural imagery of romantic love provides one essential "vocabulary of motives" that emphasizes the goals, albeit hard to realize, of caring and commitment.[27] Religious vocabularies of love and commitment provide another set of caring ideals. A religious ethic teaches us to love our neighbors as we love ourselves. To be kind, giving, altruistic, unselfish, and caring in all our relationships, but especially toward those less fortunate than ourselves, is a bedrock message of all religious groups. In America, a place with more churches and synagogues per capita than any society on earth, the idea is promoted at least once a week to millions of people that it is surely their duty to care for their families, but also for the "family of man." Although Americans seem to have far more celebrities than moral heroes, we do revere Jesus Christ, Mother Theresa, and Martin Luther King as historical figures whose compassion deserves emulation. The parable of the Good Samaritan remains a religious/ cultural story that reminds us of our responsibilities to others and of the redemptive potential of human compassion.

A related language of spirituality also stresses commitment and connection. More than ever, Americans seem to be on a "collective search for identity."[28] Now, at the millennium, those millions of people browsing the psychology and self-help sections of the bookstore are just aisles away from the spirituality section where they find inspiration and instruction in their search for self. Although the search for self has, by definition, an individualistic motif to it— it is, after all, a search for *self*—seekers often find inspiration in Eastern religious texts that preach a communitarian message. It is that we can discover our selves only through connection with others. Millions of Americans are trying to incorporate into their lives the spiritual message that all things and people are part of a seamless web, that independence is an illusion, and that spiritual enlightenment and happiness depend less on self-reliance than on mutual alliances. In a message that contradicts our notion of rugged individualism, we learn that selflessness is the only route to self-realization. It seems safe to conclude that people are drawn to spiritual, religious, and communitarian messages because they have an inchoate feeling that a life committed to self-enhancement has not been a recipe for satisfaction and happiness.

Let me offer one more example that illustrates our longing to embrace a more communal and caring ethic. For over a year, a book entitled *Tuesdays with Morrie* topped the bestseller lists.[29] The book touches me in a very particular way since I knew Morrie Schwartz, whose death the book chronicles. Morrie was special because he was able to turn his dying process from Lou Gehrig's disease into a celebration of love, connection, and community. When he learned of his terminal illness, Morrie did not withdraw from the world, as is the usual case. Rather, he created a community in his home filled with family and many friends, drawn to his bedside by Morrie's extraordinary openness and humanity, even as his death relentlessly approached.[30] Morrie's death mirrored his life. Both his personal life and public teachings as a sociology professor centered on the importance of community and care. The millions of people who learned of Morrie on Ted Koppel's *Nightline* and subsequently have read about him are moved by his story because of what they already suspect, but often cannot act on—the route to self-discovery and personal fulfillment is through community and commitment.

The cultural languages of religion, love, and spirituality incline Americans toward relationships of caring and commitment instead of self-absorption. In one realm of our lives, however, these messages are hardly necessary. Whatever influence the ethic of individualism has had in directing the *public* lives of Americans, a modified set of cultural expectation circumscribes the *private* realm of the family. Although ideas about self-expression and a life dedicated to self-enhancement have surely influenced the American family, it is the one institution that has been relatively insulated and exempted from the widely shared belief that one should consider one's own welfare before that of any social group. Moreover, if the bonds of blood are thought to supersede an individual's wishes and needs, this is most especially true for women.

In a culture otherwise dedicated to expressive individualism, women—mothers in particular—often measure their morality through an ethic of care and a willingness to subordinate self-interest to the greater good of the family. The privatizing and "engendering" of care within the family is not a cultural accident. It is the structural analogue of America's *political decision* not to bear responsibility for all the groups and individuals in need of care. In contrast to Scandinavian societies, for example, that have chosen to place the responsibility for the welfare of individuals squarely within the domain of government, the United States is groping for some consistency in the way that the poor, the ill, and the dispossessed should be cared for. As a society, we cannot agree whether individuals ought to care for themselves, whether it is primarily the family's responsibility, or whether it is ultimately society's duty to care for the less fortunate. Our economy is mixed, our cultural motives are mixed, our social sentiments are mixed, and, consequently, many of us are mixed up.

Taking Care: Whose Problem Is It Anyway?

The way that the sixty people interviewed for this study tried to answer the question "What do I owe to a mentally ill family member?" cannot be separated from the way American society, as embodied in its social programs, has decided what it owes to its members in all kinds of trouble; whether or not it will care for those who, for whatever reason, cannot care for themselves. The caregiving difficulties faced by individuals on a daily basis are intimately connected with the political decisions about who deserves help and care and what institutions will be set up to provide it. Indeed, the most heated policy debates in the United States are about care. What kinds of government provisions will be made for Americans beneath the poverty line? What kind of welfare support will be provided for our unemployed? What shall we do to help our homeless? What kind of medical benefits will we extend to the elderly? How much aid shall we provide to single mothers with dependent children? And so on.

The social structures we create are a reflection of our cultural values. It is, therefore, not terribly surprising that our society, rooted in the cherished values of rational self-interest and profit maximization, has opted not to care very much for its citizens. It's

my personal judgment that, although America's version of capitalism has produced unbelievable wealth for some, we are in a period
of unparalleled governmental uncharitability. In the same society
that pays certain athletes up to $250,000 a week to hit baseballs,
more than 25 percent of the children in America go to bed hungry.[31]
Rather than being appalled that less than 1 percent of the population owns between 20 and 25 percent of all wealth in America, such
concentration of income, stocks, bonds, and real estate in the hands
of so few is often applauded as reflecting the glory of a free-market
economy.[32] Al, a custodian and one of the people I interviewed for
Speaking of Sadness, viscerally understands marginality and its consequences. In explaining his emotional difficulties, he told me

> A big thing about depression in the United States is a lack of a sense
> of community . . . we aren't a people. We are a collective . . . and no-
> body feels like they owe anyone. . . . It's like a tough shit society. You
> know, if you're homeless, tough shit. If you get AIDS, tough shit.
> They say in England "I'm all right, Jack." You know, "I've got mine,
> Jack." And to that degree I find the United States a pretty uncivilized
> society. There is just a dreadful shallowness that promotes socio-
> pathic thinking in even normal people.

To use Al's indelicate, but accurate phrase, we need to ask just
how a "tough-shit" society affects the architecture of the American
family. The family, like every institution in a society, mirrors broad
cultural values and is deeply shaped by them. If a society has made
its choice not to step in when a person needs help, the burden
placed on family members to pick up the slack is dramatically increased. At this point in our history, we have decided that when a
person is troubled and somehow cannot manage life, it is up to
family members to struggle with the problem as best they can. We
have privatized human problems by expecting families to solve
them, largely out of public view. It is an extraordinary burden to
place on a few individuals whose culture also provides mixed messages about commitment to self and to others. Reliance on the

family creates a kind of cultural double whammy. Family members are expected to carry the moral burden of being primary caregivers in a culture that is, at the least, ambivalent about caring. They need to care enough to avoid the stigma of abandoning injured kin, but cannot care so much that they compromise their own aspirations and identities.

To understand how family members, women in particular, have come to assume the greatest share of the burden to care whenever a family member is somehow incapacitated, we need to appreciate the social forces that have shaped the family's evolution. As my earlier discussion in this chapter intimated, the family, like every social institution, was profoundly altered as America moved into the industrial age. In a book whose title well sums up his thesis, Richard Sennett has described middle-class *Families Against the City* during the latter part of the nineteenth century.[33] His historical analysis details the gradual retreat of the family and its members from the public sphere. The family became a refuge from the rigors of the industrial city and was increasingly relied on to provide a person's most meaningful face-to-face connections. Whereas the family had previously been an integral part of the larger community, it increasingly became one's whole community. "The home had . . . become the focus for a new kind of intense family life, a life that was private and isolated."[34]

The desire of middle-class families to live outside cities and the definition of the home as a haven from the turbulence of urban life must be viewed in terms of still larger symbolic processes accompanying industrialization—the sacralization of family life and the emergence of a "cult of domesticity." Historians agree that one of the most profound changes of the industrialization process was the separation of work and home. Industrial capitalism fundamentally altered the rhythm of daily life in that men traveled to work each day, leaving women behind and responsible for everything connected with home life. This was the beginning of a distinctive bifurcation of society into a male-dominated work sphere and female-dominated home sphere. Women came to be defined as sacred figures of sorts whose role stood outside the newly emerging economic system, whose personal services as wife and mother were beyond price. Such a definition led to the current situation in which women's work at home is detached from its true economic value allowing, in turn, the distinction between wage labor and domestic labor.

During the latter part of the nineteenth century, women's worlds became isolated and separated from the public sphere. Such a split contributed to the hardening of male and female roles and to the definition of home as a "haven in a heartless world."[35] The industrialization of labor fostered a celebration of the domestic role of women and a reawakening of the Anglo-Saxon view of a *man's home* as his castle. It was in the context of the changed meaning of work and women's roles that a single-family dwelling came to be "the most visible signal of having arrived at a fixed place in society, the goal to which every decent family aspired. . . . The notion of life in a private house represented stability, a kind of anchor in the heavy seas of urban life."[36] The notion of home as haven implied a commitment to privacy rather than to community:

> By 1870 separateness had become essential to the identity of the suburban house. The yard was expected to be large and private . . . in direct antithesis to the dense lifestyle from which many families had recently moved. The new ideal was no longer to be part of a close community, but to have a self-contained unit, a private wonderland walled off from the rest of the world. Although visually open to the street, the lawn was a barrier—a kind of verdant moat separating the household from the threats and temptations of the city.[37]

My brief historical excursion provides at least a partial answer to why the family has come to be seen as the "natural" locus for dealing with those who cannot function on their own and why women disproportionately shoulder the burdens of caregiving. The latter issue of the gender division of caregiving labor is, of course, a hot-button matter in American society. The question of why women "care more" provokes intense discussion, especially among feminist writers, because it calls forth different explanations for understanding the social roles of women.[38] As in many areas of social life, explanations for why people perform the social roles they do carry weighty symbolic and political significance. For example, if we (individually and as a society) are persuaded that woman are somehow biologically inclined to feel greater concern, sympathy, compassion, and care than men, it becomes, many fear, an argument for maintaining the cult of domesticity and the continued oppression of women. Equally, the way we look at and evaluate the meanings of caring is surely related to who does it, why they do it, and how they are rewarded for the effort.

Because women have traditionally done the bulk of the caregiving work within the context of highly privatized families, caring has come to be culturally devalued in quite the same way that most of women's domestic labor is taken for granted and accorded little respect. It is a related inequity that, despite their extraordinary importance to our individual and collective well-being, such traditionally female and caring professions as nursing and teaching are at the lower ends of the professional prestige hierarchy. History has set in motion a process that relegates caregiving to the private domain of family life, sees it as largely the natural moral obligation of women to accomplish, and devalues it as an activity. As a consequence, those who must make policy decisions about whether to provide institutional supports outside the family to help people in great need are not inclined to do it. Each time policy makers refuse welfare to those in desperate situations, a still greater burden is placed on already frail families. It is a vicious and inhumane cultural circle of the worst sort. Suzanne Gordon makes a similar point with the following observation:

> Corporate leaders and politicians will never give men and women time off to care for others if they think that caring is simpleminded head patting and good listening. If this traditional masculine disrespect and disdain for such activities continues unabated—even

among women—we will never convince politicians and taxpayers to allocate funds for institutional services and desperately needed support for community and family based caregiving.[39]

In recent years, we have increasingly heard the traditional values of personal responsibility and self-reliance invoked as the basis for reducing the role of government in caring for needy citizens.[40] Such arguments are more easily made when the family is seen as the primary safety net for people in personal crisis. It's easier to say that individuals who are dispossessed, sick, or otherwise needy should be primarily responsible for themselves when their families will be there to care should their circumstances utterly deteriorate. Thus, whenever politicians and others talk the language of strengthening family values, a goal that seems so completely laudable, a less visible, but pernicious agenda is to push off onto the family certain obligations that arguably belong to the government.

Underneath our public policies and ideologies about caring is the notion that family ties are qualitatively different from any others. It is a widely shared idea that the sense of obligation family members feel toward each other is merely the expression of a natural affinity, sympathy, compassion, and affection that people related by blood feel for each other. Many accept the idea, virtually without thinking, that family ties exist as they do because they are the inevitable expression of human nature. A closely aligned argument explains the sanctity of the family and altruistic care for an ailing parent, spouse, child, or sibling as consistent with God's laws. Given such assumptions, government policies that see families as the ultimate repository of care are often thought simply to reflect the rightful role of the family in the scheme of nature. However, such an idyllic and moralistic view of the family just does not square with the facts of family life, past or present. Although writing primarily about British families, Janet Finch's conclusions seem applicable to the United States. Her wide-ranging and exhaustive study of family practices leads her to conclude that

> Support between kin is important to many people . . . but it does
> not operate [according] to the kind of fixed rules implied by the
> idea that caring is "naturally" part of family relationships. In par-
> ticular, the idea, promoted by various governments, that the family
> should be the first port of call for people who need some assistance,
> does not align with what happens in practice. . . . In reality, the
> "sense of obligation" which marks the distinctive character of kin
> relationships is nothing like its image in political debate, where it
> appears as a set of ready-made moral rules, which all right-thinking
> people accept and put into practice. It is actually much less reliable
> than that. It is nurtured and grows over time between some indi-
> viduals more strongly than between others, and its practical conse-
> quences are highly variable.[41]

My impulse as a sociologist, as I hope the tone of my comments
makes clear, is to say that the caregiving must be understood within
the contexts of history, cultural values, and the immediate circumstances of people's lives. We will never resolve debates about
whether women are somehow "hardwired" to be more caring,
whether sentiments between family members are unique, or
whether the family should be accorded a status unlike any other
social institution. However, I side with those who say that that the
distribution of caring work in the United States has far less to do
with hormones, nature, or God than with historical legacies and
structural arrangements that have become hardened over time and
now seem to us as timeless. I agree with Peter Berger and Thomas
Luckmann who theorize that social reality should not be considered
a "thing" existing objectively "out there" in the world.[42] Rather,
reality is something that human beings continually negotiate, rec-
reate, alter, and disagree on. Reality is the product of political processes through which individuals and groups vie to have *their* version of reality become accepted as *the* reality for everyone.

The line of discussion pursued in the last few pages applies to
the way we respond to a wide array of human beings in need. The
view of the family as the ultimate repository of care circumscribes

the relationship between people in all kinds of trouble and the individuals who feel obliged to care for them. Family caregivers for those incapacitated by any catastrophic illness or disability no doubt feel confusion and ambivalence of the sort described by the people I interviewed. Indeed, we would not even speak of moral obligations if human choices about caring were completely unproblematic. However, as I have maintained throughout, the case of mental illness poses distinctive interpretive difficulties for the ill themselves, for those who love them, and for those who must create social policy about their care. Ambivalence about caring for the mentally ill is heightened in a society unsure about the status of mental illness itself.

Caring for the Mentally Ill

Illnesses can never be separated from social context; they are never independent of social norms and cultural values. The history of AIDS is a recent example. One of the particularly unfortunate, but predictable, features of the AIDS epidemic is that for many years little government or public concern was shown about the disease because it was viewed as largely the problem of homosexuals.[43] The lack of government response affirms that attitudes about illnesses have a strong ideological and moral component. Even after AIDS crossed over into the heterosexual population and began to infect millions of "respectable" people, large numbers of Americans persisted in feeling that those who fell victim to a sexually transmitted disease were only getting what they deserved because of their "immoral" behavior. Although suffering from the same virus, hemophiliacs who contracted AIDS through blood transfusions have been accorded a different moral status as "innocent" victims. In a similar way, those who suffer from mental illness must contend both with a horrible disease and the still negative meanings attached to it by society.

The genealogy of mental illness has not been a happy one. In his sweeping history of the cultural consciousness that has surrounded "madness," Michel Foucault shows how the asylum was invented to remove from social view those whose behaviors were seen as polluting social and moral order.[44] Histories like Foucault's also document unthinkable treatments done in the name of humanity, science, and psychiatric medicine. The mentally ill have, at different moments in history, been subject to castration, involuntary incarceration, bloodletting, brutal "electric shock" treatments, mind-numbing drugs inducing permanent neurological damage, and a variety of brain surgeries. One might think that nearly three centuries after the "Enlightenment" in Europe, mental illness would have emerged from the shadows of ignorance, fear, and stigma. Although increased public discussion in the United States, even over the last decade or so, has generated greater awareness of mental illness, sufferers and their families are still left to deal with this "unspeakable" problem largely on their own.

Along with the fear always accompanying the inexplicable, those suffering from mental illness are often shunned because of their unpredictable, confusing, frightening, and sometimes threatening behaviors. The fear, bewilderment, and anger generated by mental illness are deeply embedded in our language. When a person says or does something that we consider objectionable or incomprehensible, we angrily question their sanity. Everyday conversation is filled with derisive references to those who are "crazy," "nuts," "off their rockers," or "out of their minds." Although advocates for the mentally ill repeatedly point out that someone diagnosed with a mental illness is statistically less likely to commit a violent crime than those in the population at large, newspapers routinely stir up fear with grisly stories of crimes committed by deranged persons. Despite a number of antistigma campaigns, the public's view of mental illness may be most influenced by the media attention given to the likes of Jeffrey Dahmer or Ted Kozinski.

A distinctive problem in thinking about mental illness is that no one can judge with any confidence where normal behavior ends and disease begins, when people's mental and emotional functioning is so impaired that they truly suffer from a disease and, therefore, should not be held responsible for their behaviors. The unwillingness to see mental illness as a legitimate disease is evident in our legal system. In one highly visible trial after another, defendants, no matter how obviously disconnected from conventional reality, are judged responsible for their crimes and sent to prisons instead of hospitals. Only on rare occasions does the insanity defense succeed in court. We may acknowledge that mental illness is real, but we have trouble identifying it and even more trouble excusing behavior because of it.

Although it is never quite clear whether social science writing generates new social consciousness or merely reflects already existing cultural ideas, there is little doubt about the influence of the so-called "antipsychiatry movement" that flourished particularly during the 1960s and 1970s. Writers like Erving Goffman, Thomas Szasz, Ronald Laing, and Thomas Scheff argued that mental illness was nothing more than an arbitrary political label.[45] They saw the mental illness diagnosis as part of a sweeping "medicalization" process that increasingly deemed troublesome behaviors as diseases.[46] Mental illness, they argued, was a label attached to those whose behaviors were objectionable, troublesome, or nonconforming. Such persons, they acknowledged, might very well have significant "problems with living," but the scientific warrant for defining them as diseased simply did not exist.

These critiques of psychiatry had merit. It remains true, I think, that much of what we call mental illness is nothing more than a political designation sold as science.[47] At the same time, antipsychiatry theorists undercut their credibility by taking their argument too far. To flatly claim that mental illness does not exist seems nonsensical when persons are catatonic, visibly psychotic, or otherwise unable to understand or carry out even the most rudimentary behaviors necessary to function in a society. The stories I have heard during many years of interviewing, some of them retold in earlier chapters, persuade me that, while we do not know with any precision what abnormality occurs in people's brains and why, mental illness is, indeed, real and not just the product of overzealous labeling.

However one thinks about the ontological status of mental illness, few would defend the inhumanity of mental hospitals that largely warehoused the sickest patients prior to the 1970s. Along with the social science ethnographies that have been done over the years describing the deplorable conditions and dehumanizing character of so many mental hospitals, America's consciousness was also raised by such documentaries as *Titicutt Follies* that portrayed the brutally awful conditions in a Massachusetts state hospital during the 1960s. So, when such antipsychotic drugs as Thorazine made deinstitutionalization possible, it seemed like a moment of liberation for the mentally ill. Few could mourn the passing of a mental health hospital system that largely relegated patient care to untrained staff, too often created a context for abuse rather than genuine help, and might overall have exacerbated patients' illnesses. However, once the hospital system collapsed, patients fell into an institutional vacuum.

Along with the discovery of new psychotropic medications that insulated patients from their worst psychotic episodes, the deinstitutionalization process was hastened by the antipsychiatry movement and legislation supporting the development of community mental health centers that would presumably serve the needs of ex-patients. Based on a somewhat romantic view of the community, similar to President George Bush's call a few years ago for a "thousand points of light" to solve complicated social problems, the hope was that community mental health centers would provide necessary support to ex-patients while safeguarding their civil liberties. Although the centers established did provide modest doses of psychotherapy and life skills training, the programs were poorly supervised by the federal government, frequently degenerated because of internal politics, and failed to reach those most in need of service— the most severely and chronically ill ex-patients.

Today, community support for the mentally ill is constituted by a patchwork of diverse programs based on different assumptions about the needs of chronically ill persons. Clubhouses, halfway houses, and a variety of training programs are well-intentioned efforts to help, but lack bureaucratic regularity, therapeutic coherence, and consistent funding. In the absence of adequate public policies, the mentally ill and their families have largely been left to fend for themselves. Rather than finding sufficient community support, thousands of ex-patients live, socially isolated, in cheap single-room occupancy hotels or, worse, become part of America's burgeoning homeless population. The remaining tens of thousands retreat behind the closed doors of family homes where they remain out of the public's view and mind. The family has once again become the social institution of choice to provide care. In effect, community support has come to mean primarily family support. Moreover, if the family has replaced doctors, social workers, nurses, and the ward staff "it is a staff without shifts, without backup, without the ability to enforce daily routines or medication compliance, without techniques of rehabilitation."[48]

Underlying much of the complexity and frustration of caregiving is the difficult question of patients' rights. Certainly, the antipsychiatry movement that hastened the closing of ineffective and repressive institutions also heightened awareness about abuses of patients' civil rights. The subsequent emergence of multiple and increasingly powerful patient rights groups has enabled legislation that now makes involuntary treatment of mentally ill persons extremely difficult. Although I generally welcome laws that protect weak and vulnerable populations from the potential excesses of bureaucratic systems, the right of ill patients to refuse treatment also potentially harms those too sick to make reasoned judgments about their care. As some of the accounts in earlier chapters illustrate, the right to refuse treatment has also created a nightmarish situation for family caregivers. Unless it can be demonstrated that psychotic persons are a clear danger to themselves or others, they remain untreated. Even when caregivers are successful in gaining a court order requiring commitment, patients are quickly released after very brief treatment presumably "stabilizes" them. As Harriet Lefley describes it,

> Families' experiences with coercive treatment are painful, filled with
> ambivalence, and are lacking in viable options. They are faced with

an unresponsive treatment system and a legal system that places them in an adversarial posture against a loved one. . . . If an involuntary intervention is the only option, they must balance indignity to a loved one against his or her own destructive behavior, threats to themselves or others, the very real possibility of self-neglect or even death on the streets, or the criminalization of the illness. They themselves feel coerced by a system that offers inadequate resources and makes it difficult to help persons during a critical period, when they are perceived as incapable of helping themselves.[49]

The ethical questions surrounding the involuntary treatment of mentally ill persons have been comprehensively treated in a variety of sources.[50] I will only remark here that if we want to diminish the dreadful impact of mental illness on families, we need to find a legal middle ground between the absolute right of psychotic persons to refuse treatment and forced incarceration. The current standard that allows involuntary commitment only when a person is a clear danger to themselves or others is too restrictive. This criterion denies both families and catastrophically ill persons treatments that provide patients a measure of stability. The goal must be to find alternatives that optimally balance the rights of both individuals and families. Many favor a system of "outpatient commitment" as best protecting both patients and families.[51] Under a system of involuntary community commitment persons who have not met the criterion of dangerousness, but have nevertheless plainly deteriorated well beyond the point of functioning, could be required to receive medical treatment. Following hospitalization only long enough to moderate a psychotic episode, patient compliance with medical treatment would be closely supervised by community mental health workers.

While seeking a humane middle ground on the matter of civil commitment, policy makers, family members, and consumers of mental health services must also lobby for a coherent, integrated, and well-staffed system of community supports. Even those who disagree on the volatile issue of involuntary commitment mutually support a range of crisis alternatives—community teams that intervene to calm distressed individuals and their families, increased training for police who routinely deal with mentally ill persons, an expanded system of drop-in centers and respite houses for ill persons, and a cadre of professionally trained outreach workers to break the destructive cycle of chronically ill people who shuttle between hospitals and the streets. Service agencies must also reach out to families to provide continuing education and emotional support. In addition, family members need close guidance when they must deal with hospitals, insurance systems, and clinicians of all sorts. An integrated system of services focused, as far as possible, on the prevention of acute episodes of illness should be the first order of caring priorities for the mentally ill.

Caring for the Family

Although people across the political spectrum agree that the American family needs strengthening, the discussion is hampered by disagreements on what forms of family life are "normal" and "desirable." Rather than focusing on concrete proposals for supporting the multiple forms of family life that now exist in the United States, the conversation too often bogs down in disputes about the meaning of "family values" and the "appropriate" structure of family life. Whatever one's beliefs about family life, bolstering the family will require far more than lofty rhetoric about values and morality. It is too easy to blame the fragility of American families on the failure of individuals to acquire the "right" values. The bigger problem is that families have been abandoned by society to solve, on their own, the increasingly complex problems of their individual members. In applying a version of rugged individualism to the family, we have increasingly isolated an institution whose health requires the nourishment of public, social, and legislative support.

Societies that emphasize individualism accomplish a kind of social sleight of hand. When personal achievement is extolled above all else, those who fail are encouraged to believe that they have only themselves to blame. Victims of a system of institutionalized inequality are conned into blaming themselves for their state of affairs.[52] They suffer from a kind of false consciousness that prevents them from seeing how their fate is linked to society's failure in living up to the principles of democracy, fairness, and equality of opportunity. A similar blind spot leads us to blame families for their troubles. A few years ago, millions of people read John Bradshaw's claim that 96 percent of American families are "dysfunctional."[53] His message is that families are toxic environments and terribly hazardous to the health of their members. To be sure, many awful things happen within families. The question, though, is how best to understand why families unravel. Shall we chalk it up exclusively to the behaviors of bad people? Is the family somehow intrinsically flawed? Or might there be something wrong with the cultural soil in which families grow, thrive, or increasingly dissemble?

As with most big and pressing questions, no one explanation will do. However, by now, you will not be surprised by my perspective on the matter. The privatization of the family and the corresponding expectation that it deal largely on its own with every member's problem, big and small, is unreasonable.[54] The family, like any system, will simply begin to break down when too much is demanded from it, when its caring capacity is reached. Expecting family members to care for each other in a society that shows so little care and regard for the family is a prescription for pathology. It is specious and wishful thinking that individuals operating within a society dedicated to rationality, free choice, and individual achievement will easily shuck off those values once in the privacy of their homes. No American institution escapes the logic of a market economy and it is far more likely "that considerations of self interest associated with the economy will serve as moral codes within the family than that the family will serve as a moral world capable of influencing behavior in the economy."[55]

In their book, *The War Against Parents*, Sylvia Hewlett and Cornell West argue that government support for families has badly eroded over the last thirty years.[56] Shortly after WWII, as veterans returned home, new mortgage loan programs, the policies of the Federal Housing Administration, and the massive federal funding of an interstate highway program encouraged home ownership in the suburbs. Jobs were plentiful, workers were protected by robust unions, and tax incentives favored the family. Beginning in the 1970s, pro-family policies were increasingly replaced with pro-business policies and forms of "corporate welfare" that redirected government largesse away from people in need. My colleague Charles Derber, in a book aptly titled *Corporation Nation*, demolishes the fiction that American corporations are private enterprises. He writes that "as business leaders and politicians rhapsodize about the virtues of privatization, corporations have grown so dependent on public provision that the whole corporate system would collapse without it."[57] Through a range of government subsidies, loan guarantees, tax breaks, and tax loopholes "corporations collect more government handouts than all of the nation's poor combined."[58]

Earlier in this chapter I remarked on the writings of nineteenth-century theorists who were concerned with the weakening of social ties as societies modernized. Among them, a sociologist named Georg Simmel presciently argued that "a money economy and the dominance of the intellect are intrinsically connected."[59] In emerging capitalist economies, Simmel wrote, the individual increasingly "reacts with his head instead of his heart."[60] While Simmel's prediction generally rings true, we should not conclude that rationality thoroughly supersedes emotionality when it comes to caring for an ill family member. A more accurate description, based on the interviews in this book, is that family caregivers struggle to reconcile the conflicting demands of head and heart.

In this last chapter I have tried to understand, in terms of divergent cultural messages, the kind of ambivalence family members feel in drawing caregiving boundaries. Such ambivalence, I maintain, is predictable in a society that offers confusing messages about obligations to self and others, devalues caring work, privatizes family life, and increasingly withdraws structural support from a system already dramatically overloaded with obligations. Some observers are chagrined by the erosion of family life and find remarkable the sort of callousness that too often describes family relationships. What seems far more remarkable to me is the extraordinary reservoir of love, caring, and connection that holds families together, even at a time when family life is so meagerly supported. The data presented throughout this book testify that habits of the heart are exceedingly hard to break. However, as strong as they are, the bonds of love, caring, and commitment cannot by themselves sustain the family, besieged as it is by inimical cultural ideas and a government indifferent to its needs.

The fate of American families must be viewed as a national problem, and, as such, it is the responsibility of federal and state governments to intervene in revitalizing troubled families. Just as government neglect has undermined the infrastructure of the family, it will take substantial federal support to reverse long-term processes that have been contrary to the health of families and, thus, to the well-being of us all. Just as "globalization" increasingly illustrates that we live in a small and organically interconnected world, it is critical to realize that the fates of societies and families are intertwined. A coherent national policy must be constructed with the goal of saving families in trouble rather than standing by idly as they decay. Societies must care for and nourish families in order to ensure that parents, spouses, children, and siblings can extend compassionate care to each other during moments of vulnerability, crisis, and illness.

NOTES

ONE

1. There has been an enormous amount written about the very difficult role of caregiving to desperately sick people. Most of the voluminous literature on the caregiving role has focused either on the plight of professional caregivers, especially is settings such as nursing homes, or on family members who must deal with the debilitating effects of another person's physical illness. For a recent study on the demands of professional caregivers see K. Lyman, *Day In, Day Out with Alzheimer's: Stress in Caregiving Relationships* (Philadelphia: Temple University Press, 1993). For a recent example of the impossibly burdensome task of caring for a spouse with a degenerative physical illness see M. Cohen, *Dirty Details: The Days and Nights of a Well Spouse* (Philadelphia: Temple University Press, 1996).

Not surprisingly, the literature on caregiving focuses on such matters as persistent stress, lifestyle restrictions, the negative effects on family relations, financial difficulties, gender differences in the caregiver role, and the onset of health problems for the caregiver, including depression. A sampling of recent writing on these kinds of topics would include A. Boynkin and J. Winland-Brown, "The dark side of caring: Challenges of caregiving," *Journal of Gerontological Nursing* 21 (1995): 13–18; P. Krach and J. Brooks, "Identifying the responsibilities and needs of working adults who are primary caregivers," *Journal of Gerontological Nursing* 21 (1995): 41–50; M. Skaff and L. Pearlin, "Caregivers: Role engulfment and the loss of self,"

The Gerontologist 32 (1992): 656–64; R. Young and E. Kahana, "Specifying caregiver outcomes: Gender and relationship aspects of caregiver strain," *The Gerontologist* 29 (1989): 660–66; S. Zarit, P. Todd, and J. Zarit, "The subjective burden of husbands ands wives as caregivers: A longitudinal study," *The Gerontologist* 26 (1986): 260–66, and M. Stommel, C. Given, and B. Given, "Depression as an overriding variable explaining caregiver burden," *Journal of Aging and Health* 2 (1990): 81–102.

The bulk of writing on caregiving has been on such illnesses as Alzheimer's, other forms of dementia, and degenerative physical illnesses. The relatively smaller volume of research on caring for persons with mental illnesses has most primarily been about schizophrenia. The few investigations of caring for someone with depression largely focus on family dynamics. See, for example, G. Keitner et al., "Family functioning and the course of major depression," *Comprehensive Psychiatry* 28 (1987): 54–64; G. Fadden, P. Bebbington, and L. Kuipers, "Caring and its burdens: A study of the spouses of depressed people," *British Journal of Psychiatry* 151 (1987): 660–67; G. Keitner (ed.), *Depression and Families: Impact and Treatment* (Washington, DC: American Psychiatric Press, 1990); J. Coyne et al., "Living with a depressed person," *Journal of Consulting and Clinical Psychology* 55 (1987): 347–52; I Miller et al., "Depressed patients with dysfunctional families: Description and course of illness," *Journal of Abnormal Psychology* 101 (1992): 637–46. These articles, like nearly all the studies mentioned in this note largely report the statistical results of survey research data.

An exception to the nearly exclusively quantitative research on caregiving to a depressed person is the recent work of Terry Badger. See T. Badger, "Living with depression: Family members' experiences and treatment needs," *Journal of Psychosocial Nursing and Mental Health Research* 34 (1996): 21–29 and "Family members' experiences living with members with depression," *Western Journal of Nursing Research* 18 (1996): 149–71. Although valuable in outlining some elements of the "career" associated with caring for a depressed person, Badger's work is based on a very small sample and reports only on the experience of spouse caregivers.

2. K. Wolff (ed.), *The Sociology of Georg Simmel* (Glencoe, IL: The Free Press, 1950), p. 395.

3. Sociologists have long emphasized that reciprocity and exchange are among the fundamental normative underpinnings of social order. The early twentieth-century theorist Georg Simmel observed that "if every grateful action from good turns received in the past were suddenly eliminated, society would disappear." See *The Sociology of Georg Simmel* (Glencoe, IL: The Free Press, 1950; edited and translated by K. Wolff). In the 1960s a number of American sociologists offered versions of what came to be called

exchange theory. See especially G. Homans, *Human Behavior* (New York: Harcourt, Brace and World, 1961) and P. Blau, *Exchange and Power in Social Life* (New York: John Wiley, 1964).

4. K. Duff, *The Alchemy of Illness* (New York: Bell Tower, 1993), p. 83.

5. This study began with several months' observation in a support group for the family members of mentally ill people. Although I continue to attend weekly meetings, my involvement with the support group between December 1996 and May 1997 served as a preface to the interviewing stage of this study. Those several months of observation clarified domains of conversation that would be important to pursue through in-depth interviews. Thus, along with six "pilot" interviews conducted for a single chapter on caregivers in my earlier book on depression, *Speaking of Sadness* (New York: Oxford University Press, 1996), I conducted fifty-four additional in-depth interviews between May 1997 and July 1998. Twenty of the interviews were done with support group members who expressed a willingness to be interviewed. Advertisements placed in a local newspaper eventually yielded nineteen interviews. Another fifteen interviews were obtained through referrals. This book, then, is based on a total of sixty interviews. Although questions about obligation, duty, and responsibility are at the core of the research project, these matters do not exhaust the range of issues explored in the interviews that typically run between two and three hours. With the exception of the six pilot interviews, each of the additional fifty-four interviewees was asked to sign a consent form describing the goals of the study and guaranteeing confidentiality.

In order to interpret my findings, let me note that fifty-eight of the respondents are white. Of the remaining two, one is African American and the other Filipino. Using their occupations as a proxy for social class position, I can also report that 28 percent ($n = 17$) are professional workers, 20 percent ($n = 12$) are white-collar workers, 12 percent ($n = 7$) occupy clerical positions, 8 percent ($n = 5$) are blue-collar workers, 13 percent ($n = 8$) are students, and 18 percent ($n = 11$) were unemployed or retired at the time of the interview. It is also important to report that women are significantly overrepresented in the sample ($n = 40$). Among the forty women interviewed, fourteen were parents of an ill person, eight were spouses or partners, nine were children, eight were siblings, and one was a friend. The corresponding numbers for the twenty men in the sample are six parents, six spouses or partners, five children, one sibling, and two friends. The greater willingness of women to volunteer for participation in this study is consistent with their generally greater involvement in caregiving roles of all sorts.

6. It is certainly one of the most consistent findings in social science

literature that caregiving work within the context of families is highly gendered. In her exhaustive study of family obligations, *Family Obligations and Social Change* (Cambridge, UK: Polity Press, 1989), Janet Finch concludes that "without doubt variation by gender is a key element in patterns of support between kin" (p. 52). Women are most largely responsible for what Micaela Di Leonardo calls "kin work." See M. Di Leonardo, "The female world of cards and holidays: Women, families and the work of kinship," *Signs* 12 (1987): 40–53. At every point within family systems, women appear to have greater responsibility than men when care of a family member is required. For example, women constitute 75 percent of the unpaid caregivers to the elderly. See J. Waldrop, "Who are the caregivers?" *American Demographics* 11 (1989):39. For additional writing that examines the disproportionate role of women in family caregiving, see M. Devault, *Feeding the Family: The Social Organization of Caring as Gendered Work* (Chicago: University of Chicago Press, 1991); V. Olesen, "Caregiving, ethical and informal," *Journal of Health and Social Behavior* 30 (1989): 1–10; E. Abel and M. Nelson (eds.), *Circles of Care* (Albany: State University of New York Press, 1990); J. Finch and D. Groves (eds.), *A Labour of Love: Women, Work and Caring* (London, UK: Routledge and Kegan Paul, 1983); C. Gilligan, *In a Different Voice: Psychological Theory and Women's Development* (Cambridge: Harvard University Press, 1982); N. Noddings, *Caring: A Feminine Ethics and Moral Education* (Berkeley: University of California Press, 1984), and S. Gordon, P. Benner, and N. Noddings (eds.), *Caregiving: Readings in Knowledge, Practice, and Politics* (Philadelphia: University of Pennsylvania Press, 1996).

Rather than segregating a discussion of the gender differences in my sample to a single chapter, I have decided instead to integrate discussion of such differences into the text wherever it seems most appropriate. While generally supporting the findings of prior research that there is an unequal gender division of caregiving labor—both logistical and emotional labor— my materials also suggest that it would be unfair to stereotype men as somehow uninterested, unwilling, or unable to provide deeply compassionate care to a mentally ill family member. Among both the men I interviewed and those who regularly attend the family support group are several who are deeply involved in all aspects of a family member's care.

7. D. Karp, *Speaking of Sadness: Depression, Disconnection, and the Meanings of Illness* (New York: Oxford University Press, 1996).

8. M. Manning, "Invisible Wounds," *The New York Times Book Review*, January 21, 1996: 29.

9. A. Frank, *The Wounded Storyteller* (Chicago: University of Chicago Press, 1995).

10. A. Frank, *At the Will of the Body* (Boston: Houghton Mifflin, 1991).

11. A. Frank, 1995, op. cit., p. 25.

12. The extent to which one person's life narrative can be shaped by his or her association with a catastrophically sick person is demonstrated in Carolyn Ellis's book *Final Negotiations: A Story of Love, Loss, and Chronic Illness* (Philadelphia: Temple University Press, 1995). Ellis's writing blurs the boundaries of biographical narrative, literature, and sociology. It is, as advertised in the subtitle, "a story of love, loss, and chronic illness." The love story between Carolyn Ellis and Gene Weinstein begins with their meeting at SUNY Stony Brook in 1975. She was a new sociology graduate student and he a professor. The remainder of the book details, with the thickest biographical description I have ever read, the evolution of their relationship and Gene's battle with emphysema, ending with his death in 1985. The point here is that Ellis's life story became virtually indistinguishable from Gene's. Gene's story became hers and vice versa. Her whole book, in fact, is a chronicle of the inextricable interconnections of their presumably separate biographies.

13. L. Slater, *Welcome to My Country* (New York: Random House, 1996), p. 124.

14. A. Frank, 1995, op. cit., p. 98.

15. See my account of how the members of this depression self-help group construct a set of ideological beliefs about the character of their illness. The study entitled "Illness ambiguity and the search for meaning: A case study of a self-help group for affective disorders" appeared in the *Journal of Contemporary Ethnography* 21 (1992): 139–70.

16. One of the great values of systematic data collection is to show that events and circumstances that seem utterly chaotic from the point of view of the person experiencing a crisis actually play out in a predictable way. I tried to demonstrate this in *Speaking of Sadness*. Another example illustrating the order invisible to the person in the middle of a difficult life process is Diane Vaughan's book *Uncoupling: Turning Points in Intimate Relationships* (New York: Oxford University Press, 1986).

17. Examples of first-person accounts of living with mental illness would include the following: S. Plath, *The Bell Jar* (New York: Bantam, 1972); N. Mairs, *Plaintext Essays* (Tucson: University of Arizona Press, 1986); W. Styron, *Darkness Visible: A Memoir of Madness* (New York: Random House, 1990); E. Wurtzel, *Prozac Nation* (Boston: Houghton Mifflin, 1994).

18. Recent examples of memoirs of persons who have lived with a family member's mental illness include J. Neugeboren, *Imagining Robert: My*

Brother, Madness and Survival (New York: William Morrow, 1996) and C. Simon, *Mad House* (New York: Random House, 1997).

19. K. Erikson, "On sociological prose," *The Yale Review* 78 (1989): 525–38.

20. The nineteenth-century theorist Max Weber argued that a person's place within a class or stratification system deeply influenced his or her "life chances." Indeed, his writing suggests that the study of stratification was necessarily concerned with the patterned and unequal distribution of life chances within a society. See M. Weber, *The Theory of Social and Economic Organization* (New York: Oxford University Press, 1947; translated by A. M. Henderson and Talcott Parsons).

21. The theorist Georg Simmel inquired into the basis for social order when he asked the question, "How is society possible?" The question of social order is often said to be the most central underlying concern of sociology. Although Simmel raised the question of the possibility of society, the question of order is often traced to the writings of Thomas Hobbes, a seventeenth-century philosopher. See T. Hobbes, *Leviathan* (New York: Penguin Books, 1961; edited by C. B. MacPherson). An effort to provide a theoretical answer to the basis for social order underlies the writings of Talcott Parsons. See his book *Essays in Sociological Theory* (Glencoe, IL: The Free Press, 1954). It might also be said that Sigmund Freud was offering an answer to the question of order in his book *Civilization and Its Discontents* (New York: W. W. Norton, 1988).

22. C. W. Mills, *The Sociological Imagination* (New York: Oxford University Press, 1959), p. 158.

23. See, for example, R. Bellah et al., *Habits of the Heart: Individualism and Commitment in American Life* (Berkeley: University of California Press, 1985).

24. C. Derber, *The Wilding of America: How Greed and Violence Are Eroding Our National Character* (New York: St. Martin's Press, 1996) and Z. Bauman, *Mortality, Immortality, and Other Life Strategies* (Stanford: Stanford University Press, 1992).

25. R. Bogdan and S. Taylor, "Toward a sociology of acceptance: The other side of the sociology of deviance," *Social Policy* (Fall 1987), p. 34. Along these same lines see R. Bogdan and S. Taylor, "Relationships with severely disabled people: The social construction of humanness," *Social Problems* 36 (April, 1989): 135–48.

26. J. Neugeboren, *Imagining Robert: My Brother, Madness and Survival.* (New York: William Morrow, 1996), p. 278.

TWO

1. The general perspective guiding my analysis throughout this book is called "symbolic interaction theory." The most essential idea of this theoretical perspective is that nothing in the world—no object, event, or situation—has any intrinsic meaning. Rather, meaning is bestowed on everything by human beings. The social world is a product of people's definitions and interpretations of it. Human beings, through communication with each other, define the meaning of everything. In this regard, all human experience is an ongoing exercise in sense-making. In his book *Symbolic Interaction: Perspective and Method* (Englewood Cliffs, NJ: Prentice-Hall, 1969), Herbert Blumer articulates the three most general premises of symbolic interaction theory. They are:

1. Human beings act toward things or situations on the basis of the meanings that the things or situations have for them.
2. These meanings are derived from or arise out of the social interaction individuals have with others.
3. These meanings are handled or modified through the interpretive process used by individuals in dealing with the things or situations they encounter.

In every chapter of this book, I am concerned with how caregivers make sense of a family member's mental illness. I want to illuminate the interpretive processes caregivers engage in as they define the character of their obligations to an ill parent, child, sibling, or spouse.

2. Among these many valuable concepts provided by Erving Goffman is the notion of "situational involvement." In his 1963 book *Behavior in Public Places* (New York: Free Press), Goffman suggests that whenever we enter a social occasion, we must, in order to appear social, proper, and worthwhile, correctly answer the question "Just what level of involvement must I have with others in this situation?" Cocktail parties, business meetings, sporting events, bedrooms, anonymous public places, and classrooms, to name a few contexts, demand very different degrees of involvement from participants. The notion of situational involvement is a guiding frame for analysis in this chapter and throughout this book. I begin with the presumption that mental illness poses distinctive involvement dilemmas for the family members of an afflicted person. How they then decide on proper levels of situational involvement is a central question here and in all the chapters.

I have previously used Goffman's notion of "situational involvement" to think about the character of interaction in college classrooms and urban public places. See D. Karp and W. Yoels, "The college classroom: Some observations on the meanings of student participation," *Sociology and Social Research* 60 (July, 1976): 421–39; D. Karp, "Hiding in pornographic bookstores: A reconsideration of the nature of urban anonymity," *Urban Life and Culture* 4 (1973): 427–51. See also Chapter 4, "The social organization of everyday city life," in D. Karp, G. Stone, and W. Yoels, *Being Urban: A Sociology of City Life* (New York: Praeger, 1991).

3. See A. Strauss, *Negotiations: Varieties, Contexts, Processes, and Social Order* (San Francisco: Jossey-Bass, 1978).

4. The idea of "joint career" comes from H. Blumer, *Symbolic Interaction: Perspective and Method* (Englewood Cliffs, NJ: Prentice-Hall, 1969).

5. See W. Kaminer, "Chances are you're co-dependent too," *New York Times Book Review* (February 11, 1990), pp. 1, 26ff. Also, M. Beattie, *Codependent No More* (San Francisco: Harper San Francisco, 1992).

6. The respondent quoted here describes her impulse to care for her mother as *natural*. It is certainly a widely held idea that caregiving, most particularly the care provided by women, arises somehow from biology, human nature, or the inevitable affinity, sympathy, compassion, or affection that family members feel for each other. However, consistent with the essential ideas of symbolic interaction theory, I will maintain throughout that the obligations and emotions associated with caring for family members are *socially profiled* rather than somehow part of the inevitable and natural order of things. Such an argument has important political implication because it challenges the notion that the current division of caregiving labor within families is somehow preordained. The fact, for example, that women do a disproportionate share of caregiving work has far more to do with historical legacies, structural arrangements, cultural conventions, and arbitrary definitions of reality than with the mandates of biology or human nature.

7. C. Clark, *Misery and Company: Sympathy in Everyday Life* (Chicago: University of Chicago Press, 1997).

8. D. Tannen, *You Just Don't Understand: Men and Women in Conversation* (New York: William Morrow, 1990).

9. C. Nippert-Eng, *Work and Home* (Chicago: University of Chicago Press, 1996), p. xi.

10. See N. Denzin, *Interpretive Biography* (Newbury Park, CA: Sage Publications, 1989).

11. E. Erikson, *Identity: Youth and Crisis* (New York: W. W. Norton, 1968).

12. B. Bettelheim, *Surviving and Other Essays* (New York: Knopf, 1979).

13. V. Frankl, *Man's Search for Meaning* (New York: Pocket Books, 1988).

14. A. Strauss, "Turning points in identity." In C. Clark and H. Robboy (eds.), *Social Interaction* (New York: St. Martin's Press, 1992).

15. C. Degler, *In Search of Human Nature* (New York: Oxford University Press, 1991).

16. The way the respondents "theorize" about the causes of a family member's mental illness will be elaborated in Chapter 5, "The Four Cs."

17. See L. Hoffman, "Empathic emotions of justice in society," *Social Justice Research* 3(1989): 283–311 and M. Lerner, "The justice motive in social behavior," *Journal of Social Issues* 31 (1975): 1–20.

18. See W. Wilson, *The Truly Disadvantaged: The Inner City, the Underclass, and Public Policy* (Chicago: University of Chicago Press, 1987).

19. See T. Parsons, *Essays in Sociological Theory* (Glencoe, IL: The Free Press, 1954).

20. See, for example, R. Collins, "On the microfoundations of macrosociology," *American Journal of Sociology* 86 (1981): 984–1014; N. Denzin, "Emotions as lived experience," *Symbolic Interaction* 8 (1984): 223–40; N. Denzin, "On understanding emotion," in T. Kemper (ed.), *Research Agendas in the Sociology of Emotions* (Albany: State University of New York Press, 1990); D. Franks (series ed.), *Social Perspectives on Emotion* (Greenwich, CT: JAI Press, 1995); R. Harré and W. Parrott (eds.), *The Emotions: Social, Cultural, and Biological Dimensions* (Thousand Oaks, CA: Sage Publications, 1996); A. Hochschild, *The Managed Heart: Commercialization of Human Feeling* (Berkeley: University of California Press, 1983); A. Hochschild, "Emotion work, feeling rules, and social structure," *American Journal of Sociology* 85 (1979): 551–75; A. Hochschild, "Ideology and emotion management: A perspective and path for future research," in T. Kemper (ed.), *Research Agendas in the Sociology of Emotions* (Albany: State University of New York Press, 1990); T. Kemper, "Social constructionist and positivist approaches to the sociology of emotions," *American Journal of Sociology* 87 (1981): 336–62; S. Schott, "Emotion and social life: A symbolic interactionist analysis," *American Journal of Sociology* 84 (1979): 1317–34.

21. Hochschild, 1973, op. cit.

22. Bellah et al., 1985, op. cit.

23. Ibid., p. 93.

24. For a discussion of the idea of the "caregiving burden," see M. Caserta, D. Lund, and S. Wright, "Exploring the caregiver burden inventory (cbi): Further evidence for a multidimensional view of burden, *International Journal of Aging and Human Development* 43 (1996): 21–34.

25. A. Frank, *At the Will of the Body* (Boston: Houghton Mifflin, 1991), p. 6.

26. Ibid., p. 47.

THREE

1. C. Clark, "Emotions and micropolitics in everyday life: Some patterns and paradoxes of 'place,' " in T. Kemper (ed.), *Research Agendas in the Sociology of Emotions* (Albany: State University of New York Press, 1990), p. 323.

2. P. Thoits, "Emotional deviance: Research agendas" in T. Kemper (ed.), *Research Agendas in the Sociology of Emotions* (Albany: State University of New York Press, 1990).

3. Although this study includes family members of persons suffering from three disorders—depression, manic-depression, and schizophrenia—it is important to point out that these three illnesses do not fall into the same general diagnostic category. Only the first two, depression and manic-depression, are considered mood or affective disorders. Schizophrenia, in contrast, is considered a thought disorder.

4. The sociology of emotions begins with the presumption that our emotions cannot be understood as noncognitive, exclusively biological phenomena. They cannot be reduced to simple physiological states. Rather, emotions are "socially constructed," linked, as they are, to the immediate contexts of interactions and broader cultural norms about "appropriate" feelings in particular situations. Through a socialization process we learn what to feel at weddings, funerals, sporting events, and so on. We learn where, when, and to what extent we can express joy, grief, anger, jealousy, and the like. Contrasts across cultures show that appropriate emotional expression in one may be thought wrong in another. In short, the way we come to feel what we do, how we evaluate our own emotions, and how we endeavor to change them must be considered in terms of explicit social norms. Some of the most significant statements on the "sociology of emotions" are listed in note 20 in Chapter 2. For a more explicit treatment of the socially structured character of emotions related to the experience of illness, see V. James and J. Gabe, *Health and the Sociology of Emotions* (Oxford, UK: Blackwell Publishers, 1996).

5. A. Hochschild, "Ideology and emotion management: A perspective and path for future research," in T. Kemper (ed.), *Research Agendas in the Sociology of Emotions* (Albany: State University of New York Press, 1990), p. 117.

6. A. Hochschild, "Emotion work, feeling rules, and social structure," *American Journal of Sociology* 85 (1979): 551–75.

7. A brand of sociology termed ethnomethodology is concerned with discovering the implicit methods, assumptions, and theories people use in

"constructing" social order. One strategy employed by ethnomethodologists to illuminate the basis for social order has been the use of so-called "breaching experiments." Breaching experiments turn on purposively behaving in ways that go against normative expectations to see how individuals then reconstruct the disrupted social order. One of the most consistent findings of these experiments is that even relatively slight breaches of social order will generate strong negative reactions. See H. Garfinkel, *Studies in Ethnomethodology* (Englewood Cliffs, NJ: Prentice-Hall, 1967).

8. See B. Glaser and A. Srauss, *Time for Dying* (Chicago: Aldine, 1968); B. Glaser and A. Strauss, *Awareness of Dying* (Chicago: Aldine, 1965).

9. D. Karp, *Speaking of Sadness: Depression, Disconnection, and the Meanings of Illness* (New York: Oxford University Press, 1996).

10. A. Strauss, "Turning points in identity," in C. Clark and H. Robboy (eds.), *Social Interaction* (New York: St. Martin's Press, 1992).

11. A. Hochschild, *The Managed Heart: Commercialization of Human Feeling* (Berkeley: University of California Press, 1983).

12. A. Hochschild, 1990, op, cit., p. 118.

13. S. Gordon, "Social structural effects on emotion," in T. Kemper (ed.), *Research Agendas in the Sociology of Emotions* (Albany: State University of New York Press, 1990), p. 164.

14. A. Hochschild, 1979, op. cit.

15. The term "anomie" has a long history in sociology. The nineteenth-century sociologist, Emile Durkheim, writing on the causes of suicide, argued that a state of anomie, or relative normlessness, arose during periods of rapid social change. When norms fall into a state of flux and society becomes "anomic," people feel less integrated into society and rates of suicide rise. See Durkheim's famous work *Suicide* (New York: Free Press, 1966). Variations of Durkheim's notion of anomie have found their way into explanations of a range of social phenomena besides suicide. One famous use of "anomie theory" was to explain various forms of deviance in society. Robert Merton argued that when a society holds out general achievement goals while not providing the means to achieve those goals for significant segments of the population, anomie will ensue. Those unable to realize success goals through legitimate social channels will find illegitimate means to achieve them. See R. Merton, "Social structure and anomie," *American Sociological Review* 3 (1938): 672–82. The term is appropriate here because, prior to a diagnosis, caregivers have no normative basis for understanding the behaviors of mentally ill family members. Thus, they experience confusion about what to feel.

16. See, T. Scheff, *Being Mentally Ill* (Chicago: Aldine, 1966); T. Szasz, *Ideology and Insanity* (Garden City, NY: Anchor Books, 1970); E. Goffman,

Asylums: Essays on the Social Situation of Mental Patients (Garden City, NY: Doubleday Anchor, 1961), and R. Laing, *The Politics of Experience* (New York: Ballantine Books, 1967).

17. See B. Thorne and Z. Luria, "Sexuality and gender in children's daily worlds," *Social Problems* 33 (1986): 176–90.

18. See M. Kimmel and M. Messner (eds.), *Men's Lives* (New York: Macmillan, 1989).

19. See A. Daniels, "Invisible work," *Social Problems* 34 (1987): 403–15.

20. The notion of "kin work" comes from M. Di Leonardo, "The female world of cards and holidays: Women, families and the work of kinship," *Signs* 12 (1987): 40–53.

21. Hochschild, 1979, op. cit.

22. The capacity to adjust one's behavior in response to particular situations was termed role-taking by the philosopher George Herbert Mead. From Mead's perspective, the development of the self is inextricably bound up with the capacity to take the role of others. Every act of role-taking simultaneously involves two dimensions: (1) persons anticipating the responses that others are going to make toward them, and (2) persons evaluating their own behaviors in terms of the anticipated responses of others. The issue of role-taking is central to my analysis since mental illness often makes mutual role-taking between caregivers and family members impossible. In everyday life, problems in role-taking generate miscommunications. That is, there is always the possibility that our attempts at role-taking will lead us to formulate a definition of the situations that varies from the definition held by those with whom we are communicating. When this happens, interactions become, at the least, problematic and may fail altogether. Mental illnesses are characterized by the inability of the sick person to role-take with "normal" people. It is the very character of such illnesses that sufferers define reality in ways that their caregivers cannot understand. For more extended discussions of the central place of role-taking for meaningful communication, see G. H. Mead, *Mind, Self, and Society* (Chicago: University of Chicago Press, 1934).

23. Individuals in a state of hypomania experience an elevated mood, feelings of elation, grandiosity, and intense well-being. Hypomania is typically associated with a decreased need for sleep and, often, with high levels of achievement. It is not surprising that people with manic-depression frequently will not comply with medication because they are unwilling to give up the experience of hypomania. However, during hypomanic periods individuals lose insight into the likelihood that hypomania typically precedes full-blown episodes of psychotic mania.

24. See D. Franks, "Power and role-taking," in D. Franks and D. Mc-

Carthy (eds.), *The Sociology of Emotion* (Greenwich, CT: JAI Press, 1989); D. Thomas, D. Franks, and J. Calanico, "Role-taking and power in social psychology," *American Sociological Review* 37 (1972): 605–15.

25. D. Thomas, D. Franks, and J. Calanico, ibid.

26. See R. Rosenthal et al., "Body talk and tone of voice: The language without words," *Psychology Today* 8 (September 1974): 64–68; D. Archer and M. Constanza, "Interpreting the expressive behavior of others: The interpersonal perception task," *Journal of Nonverbal Behavior* 13 (1989): 225–45; D. Archer and M. Constanza, *The Interpersonal Perception Task* (Berkeley, CA: University of California Extension Media Center, 1988).

27. There is also evidence that role-taking ability varies among racial groups, certainly another area of social life in which there are substantial power differentials. In one study, forty-eight undergraduate students, both blacks and whites, were presented with a set of photographs. They were then asked to choose, from a list of seven emotions, the one they believed was being expressed by the person in each picture. The results indicate that "[blacks] were superior both in terms of overall accuracy score as well as correct scores for the individual emotions" (p. 28). See G. Gitter, H. Black, and D. Mostofsky, "Race and sex in the communication of emotion," *Journal of Social Psychology* 88 (1972): 273–76. Data on the relationship between race and role-taking ability are still quite limited and little has been done since the Gitter et al. study. In addition, most studies examining racial differences in nonverbal behaviors have failed to control for respondents' socioeconomic status, so it is not at all clear what accounts for such differences. See S. Manstead, "Expressiveness as an individual difference," in R. Feldman and B. Rime (eds.), *Fundamentals of Nonverbal Behavior* (New York: Cambridge University Press, 1991).

28. Elaboration of the idea of the "sick role" is found in T. Parsons, *Essays in Sociological Theory* (Glencoe, IL: The Free Press, 1954).

29. C. Clark analyzes the distribution and expression of sympathy as part of an "emotional economy" in her book *Misery and Company: Sympathy in Everyday Life* (Chicago: University of Chicago Press, 1997).

30. I have already commented on the way that women are socialized to assume a greater involvement than men when family members need care. It follows that when persons outside the family perceive that a sick person is not being well cared for, blame is far more likely to be directed at women than at men. Women are, therefore, often twice penalized. They are expected to do most of the caregiving and are then too often criticized by onlookers who do not understand the unique caregiving problems associated with mental illness.

31. C. W. Mills, *The Sociological Imagination* (New York: Oxford University Press, 1959), p. 4.

FOUR

1. The conventional wisdom in the social sciences is that the capacity to generalize from studies with relatively small samples is limited. Most research methods textbooks maintain that firm generalizations require large samples of respondents who are chosen through processes of random selection. For this reason, small sample in-depth interview studies like this one are often judged to have limited generalizabilty. While I certainly agree that "statistical" generalizations of the sort generated by survey research studies require large samples, there is another sort of generalization possible from relatively small sample studies like this one. I make the distinction between "empirical" and "analytical" generalizations. Empirical generalizations are of the sort made in large-scale survey research studies in which the goal is to generalize from a "representative sample" of people to a larger "universe" of individuals. In contrast, the theorist Georg Simmel argued that the goal of sociological research ought to be the discovery of generic, underlying "forms" of social life. In this study, for example, my goal is to reveal the social forms of obligation and responsibility to an ill family member. Although it is always important to consider the limitations of any sample, I maintain that the discovery of such underlying and patterned dimensions to social life is best realized through the kind of qualitative, in-depth data reported on in this volume. For a fuller discussion of the goals of a "formal sociology," see G. Simmel, "The study of social forms," in K. Wolff (ed.), *The Sociology of Georg Simmel* (Glencoe, IL: The Free Press, 1950).

2. See, for example, C. Charmaz and D. Paternini (eds.), *Health, Illness, and Healing* (Los Angeles: Roxbury Publishing Company, 1999); P. Conrad (ed.), *The Sociology of Health and Illness* (New York: St. Martin's Press, 1997).

3. Shabbot refers to the Friday evening dinner prior to the Jewish day of Sabbath that is observed on Saturday.

4. The notion that the order of everyday life rests on a set of taken-for-granted assumptions is especially developed in the philosophical writings of Alfred Schutz. See A. Schutz, *Collected Papers: Studies in Social Theory* (The Hague: Martinus Nijhoff, 1960).

5. See J. Clair, D. Karp, and W. Yoels, *Experiencing the Life Cycle: A Social Psychology of Aging* (Springfield, IL: Charles Thomas, 1993).

6. See, for example, B. Neugarten, J. Moore, and J. Lowe, "Age norms, age constraints, and adult socialization," *American Journal of Sociology* 70 (1965): 710–17.

7. A. Hochschild, *The Managed Heart: Commercialization of Human Feeling* (Berkeley: University of California Press, 1983).

8. T. Bottomore and M. Rubel (eds.), *Karl Marx: Selected Writings in Sociology and Social Philosophy* (London: C.A. Watts, 1956).

9. The notion of an "obligation hierarchy" is discussed in J. Finch, *Family Obligations and Social Change* (Cambridge, UK: Polity Press, 1989).

10. In the book that first really introduced Prozac to America, Peter Kramer describes how the diagnosis of mental illness often turns on the way patients respond to drugs. If, after taking Prozac, a person feels less melancholy, this is seen as evidence that depression is a proper diagnosis. In other words, rather than treatments being contingent on diagnoses, it is the response to treatment that often determines the diagnosis. This is especially likely in diagnosing psychiatric illness. The direction of causality from drug reaction to diagnosis is captured in the title of Kramer's book, *Listening to Prozac* (New York: Viking, 1993).

FIVE

1. Beginning with Harold Garfinkel's book *Studies in Ethnomethodology* (Englewood Cliffs, NJ: Prentice-Hall, 1967), a group of sociologists who called themselves ethnomethodologists sought to redirect the focus of sociological work. The word "ethnomethodology" referred to the study of the practical methodologies employed by everyday people. In a challenge to conventional sociological analysis, Garfinkel wrote that "Although sociologists take socially structured scenes of everyday life as a point of departure they rarely see, as a task of sociological inquiry in its own right, the general question of how any such commonsense world is possible" (p. 36). Ethnomethodologists made the same point on which this chapter turns. It is that all human beings are theorists, although they don't think of their perceptions of the world this way. That being the case, sociology should be centrally concerned with discovering the implicit theories of human actors that make possible a sense of social life as ordered, as something we can take for granted.

2. When I first discovered the MDDA group nearly ten years ago, I began attending meetings with two agendas in mind. First, I sought support because of my own problems with depression. However, I also attended meetings as a sociologist who wanted to make sense of what went on in

the groups. One of the first things I wrote on depression was an analysis of the "illness ideologies" that seemed evident in the collective discussions of depressed individuals. My analysis of the group conversation can be found in a paper entitled "Illness ambiguity and the search for meaning: A case study of a self-help group for affective disorders," *Journal of Contemporary Ethnography* 21 (1992): 139–70.

3. See C. W. Mills, "Situated actions and vocabularies of motive," in J. Manis and B. Meltzer (eds.), *Symbolic Interaction* (Boston: Allyn and Bacon, 1972).

4. P. Rieff, *Triumph of the Therapeutic* (New York: Harper and Row, 1966).

5. As several cultural observers have noted, the behavior of individuals in today's society are dominated by "experts." As an example, see C. Derber, W. Schwartz, and Y. Magrass, *Power in the Highest Degree: Professionals and the Rise of a New Mandarin Class* (New York: Oxford University Press, 1990). Experts advise us on virtually every aspect of our lives. Today, experts follow us through the life course. They are there when we are born and follow us each step along the way, eventually to our graves. Many have come to feel reliant on experts to tell them how to maintain their health, how to become educated, and how to raise their children. In his book entitled *Profession of Medicine* (New York: Dodd, Mead, 1970), Eliot Freidson indicates the enormously expanded role of professionals in our daily lives with his comment that "the relation of the expert to modern society seems in fact to be one of the central problems of our time, for at its heart lie the issues of democracy and freedom and the degree to which ordinary men can shape the character of their own lives" (p. 336).

6. M. Beattie, *Codependent No More: How to Stop Controlling Others and Start Caring for Yourself* (San Francisco: Harper San Francisco, 1992).

7. T. Moore, *Care of the Soul* (New York: HarperCollins, 1992), pp. 18–19.

8. See S. Kirk and H. Kutchens, *The Selling of DSM: The Rhetoric of Science in Psychiatry* (New York: Aldine DeGreuter, 1992) and P. Caplan, *They Say You're Crazy: How the World's Most Powerful Psychiatrists Decide Who's Normal* (Reading, MA: Addison-Wesley, 1995).

9. A renaissance in biological thinking has stirred debate about such matters as human intelligence. Among the most hotly debated books in the last few years has been Richard Herrnstein's and Charles Murray's *The Bell Curve: Intelligence and Class Structure in American Life* (New York: Free Press, 1994). Herrnstein and Murray argue that the consistently lower scores of African Americans on standardized intelligence tests reflects genetic differences in the populations studied. Their thesis has been hotly contested

by those who fault the assumptions underlying their statistical analyses. The extent of the debate is no doubt related to the high visibility of *The Bell Curve* and its political ramifications. Whatever might be Hernstein's and Murray's intentions, critics point out the racist implications of their argument. As examples of the kind of discussion raised in academic circles about *The Bell Curve,* see R. Jacoby and N. Glauberman (eds.), *The Bell Curve Debate: History, Documents, Opinions* (New York: Times Books, 1995) and S. Fraser (ed.), *The Bell Curve Wars: Race, Intelligence, and the Future of America* (New York: Basic Books, 1995).

10. See L. Eisely, *Darwin's Century: Evolution and the Men Who Discovered It* (Garden City, NY: Doubleday, 1958).

11. Margaret Mead was especially influential in making the findings of anthropologists available well beyond the discipline and fostering the view that culture was more significant than biology in shaping human destiny. Among her most famous books was *Coming of Age in Samoa* (New York: William Morrow, 1961).

12. See S. Barondes, *Mood Genes: Hunting for the Origins of Mania and Depression* (New York: W. W. Freeman, 1998).

13. J. Harris, *The Nurture Assumption: Why Children Turn Out the Way They Do* (New York: Simon and Schuster, 1998).

14. B. Spock, *The Common Sense Book of Child and Baby Care* (New York: Pocket Books, 1946).

15. P. Slater, *The Pursuit of Loneliness* (Boston: Beacon Press, 1970), p. 68.

16. C. Cooley, *Human Nature and Social Order* (New York: Schocken, 1964).

17. M. Devault, *Feeding the Family: The Social Organization of Caring as Gendered Work* (Chicago: University of Chicago Press, 1991), p. 11.

18. Ibid., p. 13. See also J. Gubrium and J. Holstein, *What Is Family?* (Mountain View, CA: Mayfield, 1990). Gubrium and Holstein show how the "family," normally understood as a natural form of life, is, rather, the product of a social construction process rooted in the everyday communications and behaviors of its members.

19. A. Gramsci, *Selections from the Prison Notebooks* (New York: International Publishers, 1980).

20. R. O'Connor, *Undoing Depression: What Therapy Doesn't Teach You and Medication Can't Give You* (Boston: Little, Brown, 1997), p. 54.

21. L. Slater, *Prozac Diary* (New York: Random House, 1998).

22. Ibid., pp. 115–16.

23. For a complete discussion of the logic of analytic induction see

B. Glaser and Anselm Strauss, *The Discovery of Grounded Theory* (Chicago: Aldine, 1967).

24. D. Papolos and J. Papolos. *Overcoming Depression* (New York: HarperCollins, 1992).

25. R. O'Connor, op. cit.

26. For examples, see K. Jamison, *An Unquiet Mind* (New York: Knopf, 1995); P. Duke, *A Brilliant Madness: Living with Manic-Depressive Illness* (New York: Bantam Books, 1992), and B. Hannon, *Agents in My Brain: How I Survived Manic Depression* (Chicago: Open Court, 1997).

27. J. Johnson, *Hidden Victims, Hidden Healers: An Eight-Stage Healing Process for Families and Friends of the Mentally Ill* (Edina, MN: Pema Publications, 1994).

28. The question of order was first systematically raised by the philosopher Thomas Hobbes in his book *Leviathan* (New York: Penguin Books, edited by C. B. MacPherson, 1961). Later, Sigmund Freud in his book *Civilization and Its Discontents* (New York: W. W. Norton, 1988) asked why human beings were willing to commit themselves to a civilization that required them to repress their most fundamental drives and energies, such as libido and aggression. Building on the writings of nineteenth-century theorists, the work of Talcott Parsons became very influential in American sociology, beginning in the 1950s. Parsons was an advocate of a theory called *functionalism* that was fundamentally concerned with understanding the basis for social order. See T. Parsons, *Essays in Sociological Theory* (Glencoe, IL: The Free Press, 1954) and *The Structure of Social Action* (New York: Free Press, 1968).

29. Philosophers such as Thomas Hobbes, John Locke, and Jean Jacques Rousseau are considered "social contract theorists."

30. In their important and much discussed critique of American culture, *Habits of the Heart*, Robert Bellah and his colleagues wryly remark that American parents are of two minds about the prospect of their children leaving home. The thought that their children will leave is difficult, but perhaps more troublesome is the thought that they might not. See R. Bellah et al., *Habits of the Heart: Individualism and Commitment in American Life* (Berkeley: University of California Press, 1985). In a recent article with two Boston College colleagues, we explore the dependence/independence relationship among twenty-three high school students who anticipated identity changes as they prepared to leave home for college. Their perceptions and choices illustrate how anxiety about leaving home requires charting a course that both maximizes independence while creating a social safety net in the event that freshly constructed identities prove inadequate for the new tasks in life. See D. Karp, L. Holmstrom, and P. Gray, "Leaving home for college:

Expectations for selective reconstruction of self," *Symbolic Interaction* 21 (1998): 253–76.

31. E. Bassoff, *Mothers and Daughters: Loving and Letting Go* (New York: Penguin Books, 1988), p. 3. It strikes me as interesting that although Bassoff is writing about the need for adolescents to break away from parents, her description applies well to the circumstances of the ill people of all ages described in this book.

32. M. Beattie, op. cit., p. 9.

33. Various books provide essentially the same estimates. See, for example, S. Blumenthal and D. Kupfer (eds.), *Suicide Over the Life Cycle: Risk Factors, Assessment, and Treatment of Suicidal Patients* (Washington, DC: American Psychiatric Press, 1990) and R. Firestone, *Suicide and the Inner Voice: Risk Assessment, Treatment, and Case Management* (Thousand Oaks, CA: Sage, 1997).

34. M. Weber, *The Theory of Social and Economic Organization* (New York: Oxford University Press, 1947).

35. F. Kafka, *The Trial* (New York: Schocken Books, 1998).

36. P. Berger and B. Berger, *Sociology: A Biographical Approach* (New York: Basic Books, 1975), p. 8.

SIX

1. See D. Rothman, "A century of failure: Health care reform in America," in P. Conrad (ed.), *The Sociology of Health and Illness* (New York: St. Martin's Press, 1997).

2. Several studies of social organizations reveal that bureaucracies often function in ways that undermine the very goals for which they were established. In one early and well-known studies, Peter Blau showed how an employment agency set up to find jobs for difficult-to-place clients failed to realize its goals because employees were evaluated in terms of their success in placing the clients. In order to look good on statistical records of performance, agency employees made little efforts to place precisely the clients the organization was meant most to serve. See P. Blau, *The Dynamics of Bureaucracy: A Study of Interpersonal Relations in Two Government Agencies* (Chicago: University of Chicago Press, 1955). My colleague at Boston College, Diane Vaughan, has analyzed how the work culture at NASA led to the greatest disaster in America's space program, the *Challenger* explosion. Her book demonstrates how well-intentioned scientists using objective data to assess "acceptable risk" created a system of rules and regulations that actually enhanced the likelihood of a launch tragedy. See D. Vaughan,

The Challenger Launch Decision: Risky Technology, Culture, and Deviance at NASA (Chicago: University of Chicago Press, 1996). These and similar studies reflect what Robert Merton years ago described as the "unintended consequences" of organizational structures. See R. Merton, *Social Theory and Social Structure* (Glencoe, IL: The Free Press, 1949).

3. The logic of presentation in this chapter is similar to that followed by Lynda Lytle Holmstrom and Anne Burgess in their several studies of rape victims. These authors were interested in describing institutional responses to rape victims. Thus, they traced the careers of rape victims from the moment they reported the crime to the police and entered the health and justice systems. Like many of the families who become part of the mental health system, Holmstrom and Burgess documented how institutional responses to rape victims worsened the problem. The impersonal and sometimes callous treatment of women traumatized by rape made them feel victimized a second time by the institutions presumably existing to protect them and treat their physical and emotional trauma. See L. Holmstrom and A. Burgess, *The Victim of Rape: Institutional Reactions* (New York: John Wiley, 1978).

4. In his book *Major Themes in Sociological Theory* (New York: David McKay Company, Inc., 1977), Calvin Larson defines anomie as "the condition of a society whose normative structure has been so attenuated that its members are not provided with sufficient information as to what their social obligations should be" (p. 244). Among the earliest uses of "anomie theory" to understand the evolution of a range of social pathologies was Emile Durkheim's analysis of suicide. See E. Durkheim, *Suicide* (New York: Free Press, 1966). See also R. Merton, "Social structure and anomie," *American Sociological Review* 3 (1938): 672–82.

5. Durkheim, ibid.

6. Despite numerous attempts to understand and predict a person's likelihood of being a danger to themselves or others, psychiatrists and other experts are unable to predict dangerousness with any measure of accuracy. In an important study on psychiatric hearings to determine whether patients should be released from institutions, Stephen Pfohl analyzed the implicit theories about potential violence and dangerousness that guided the judgments of therapeutic professionals. Pfohl demonstrates that the outcome of such hearings were built on "common sense," empirically unverified assumptions about the variables that might predict dangerousness. Professionals charged with the responsibility are no better able to predict dangerousness than laypersons who use their own commonsense theories. See S. Pfohl, *Predicting Dangerousness: The Social Construction of Psychiatric Reality* (Lexington, MA: Lexington Books, 1978).

7. See, for example, P. Brown, *The Transfer of Care: Psychiatric Deinstitutionalization and Its Aftermath* (Boston: Routledge and Kegan Paul, 1985); A. Johnson, *Out of Bedlam: The Truth About Deinstitutionalization* (New York: Basic Books, 1990), and E. Torrey, *Out of the Shadows: Confonting America's Mental Illness Crisis* (New York: John Wiley, 1997).

8. See S. Kirk and H. Kutchens, *The Selling of DSM: The Rhetoric of Science in Psychiatry* (New York: Aldine DeGreuter, 1992); P. Caplan, *They Say You're Crazy* (Reading, MA: Addison-Wesley, 1995), and P. Brown, "Diagnostic conflict and contradiction in psychiatry," *Journal of Health and Social Behavior* 28 (1987): 37–50.

9. See H. Becker, E. Hughes, and B. Geer, *Boys in White: Student Culture in Medical School* (Chicago: University of Chicago Press, 1961).

10. E. Freidson, *Profession of Medicine* (New York: Dodd, Mead, 1970), p. 336.

11. P. Rieff, *Triumph of the Therapeutic* (New York: Harper and Row, 1966).

12. C. Lasch, *Haven in a Heartless World: The Family Beseiged* (New York: Basic Books, 1977).

13. C. Lasch, "Life in the therapeutic state," *New York Review of Books* (June 12, 1980), p. 28.

14. P. Baker, W. Yoels, J. Clair, and R. Allman, "Laughter in triadic geriatric medical encounters," in D. Franks, R. Erickson, and B. Cuthbertson-Johnson (eds.), *Social Perspectives on Emotion* (Greenwich, CT: JAI Press, 1997), p. 201.

15. Ibid., p. 204.

16. L. Slater, *Welcome to My Country* (New York: Random House, 1996).

17. Students of occupations and organizational life have long been interested in the tensions between professional values, professional standards, and the imperatives of bureaucratic organizations. For example, see E. Smigel, *The Wall Street Lawyer: Professional Organization Man?* (Bloomington: University of Indiana Press, 1969); R. Hall, *Organizations: Structure, Processes, and Outcomes* (Englewood Cliffs, NJ: Prentice-Hall, 1991), and E. Krause, *Death of the Guilds: Professions, States, and the Advance of Capitalism* (New Haven, CT: Yale University Press, 1996).

18. M. Weber, *The Theory of Social and Economic Organization* (New York: Oxford University Press, 1947).

19. One of the consequences of the bureaucratization of medical work is an increased sensitivity among physicians about the way they use their time. Time has become an increasingly scarce resource for doctors. It is, therefore, not surprising that from an early point in their training, doctors are socialized to control time during interactions with patients. See

W. Yoels and J. Clair, "Never enough time: How medical residents manage a scarce resource," *Journal of Contemporary Ethnography* 23 (July 1994): 185–213.

20. See E. Shorter, *History of Psychiatry* (New York: John Wiley, 1997), and E. Valenstein, *Blaming the Brain: The Truth About Drugs and Mental Illness* (New York: Free Press, 1998).

21. See, for example, H. Lefley, *Family Caregiving in Mental Illness* (Thousand Oaks, CA: Sage, 1996) and J. Greenberg et al., "Mothers caring for an adult child with schizophrenia: The effects of subjective burden on maternal health," *Family Relations* 42 (1993): 205–11.

22. See P. Berger, *Invitation to Sociology* (Garden City, NY: Doubleday, 1963). Berger's description of the paradox of culture is well captured in two chapters in *Invitation to Sociology* entitled "Man in Society" and "Society in Man."

23. Estimates place the number of Americans without any health insurance, public or private, at between thirty-one and thirty-six million. See P. Lee, D. Soffel, and H. Luft, "Costs and coverage: Pressure toward health care reform," in P. Conrad (ed.), *The Sociology of Health and Illness* (New York: St. Martin's Press, 1997).

SEVEN

1. W. Lamb, *I Know This Much Is True* (New York: HarperCollins, 1998).

2. Ibid., pp. 280–81.

3. A. Wolfe, *Whose Keeper?: Social Science and Moral Obligation* (Berkeley: University of California Press, 1989), p. 211.

4. It is an essential assumption of Sigmund Freud's book *Civilization and Its Discontents* (New York: W. W. Norton, 1988) that societies, defined as they are by bodies of rules, require human beings to repress their most basic instincts and drives. In particular, human beings cannot give free rein to their aggressive and libidinal drives. Like Thomas Hobbes before him, Freud offers an answer to why human beings are willing to commit themselves to societies whose rules and regulations chafe against human nature. Hobbes maintained that human beings rationally decide to give up freedom to gain the security of societies governed by laws. Freud's answer is connected with his famous discussion of the Oedipus complex and the inevitability of human guilt.

5. K. Erikson, *Everything in Its Path* (New York: Simon and Schuster, 1976), p. 80.

6. Discussions of "postmodernity" dominate thinking in the humanities and social sciences these days. Although the term *postmodern* has been used in a variety of different ways that make precise definition difficult, I find Kenneth Gergen's discussion in his book *The Saturated Self: Dilemmas of Identity in Contemporary Life* (New York: Basic Books, 1991) helpful. Gergen describes the period prior to the rise of scientific thinking as *premodern*. In the premodern period religious ideas provided explanations for life's most basic mysteries. The modern period is associated with the rise of science, the scientific method, and the Newtonian idea that definitive laws about the universe could be discovered. The Newtonian imagery of modernity is that the universe is like a giant machine whose mechanisms could ultimately be understood through rational investigation. Modernity, in other words, is characterized by a belief in the possibility of discovering truth. In our current postmodern period, the notion that there are discoverable and absolute truths has come under attack. One of Gergen's chapters is titled "Truth in Trouble." Postmodernists argue that all claims to truth are really rooted in ideological ideas that, under close examination, can be "deconstructed." In the postmodern world, characterized by an explosion of information technologies, people are confronted with multiple and contradictory messages about virtually everything. In this way, postmodernity replaces faith in science with a radical relativism that undermines any claims to truth. Gergen writes that "under postmodern conditions, persons exist in a state of continuous construction and reconstruction; it is a world where anything goes that can be negotiated. Each reality of self gives way to reflexive questioning, irony, and ultimately the playful probing of yet another reality" (p. 7).

7. The communitarian ethos is spelled out in A. Etzioni, *The Spirit of Community: The Reinvention of America Society* (New York: Simon and Schuster, 1993) and in A. Etzioni (ed.), *The Essential Communitarian Reader* (Lanham, MD: Rowman and Littlefield Publishers, 1998).

8. F. Tönnies, *Fundamental Concepts of Sociology* (New York: American Book Company, 1940, translated and supplemented by Charles F. Loomis).

9. Ibid., p. 74.

10. Etzioni, 1993, op. cit., p. 18.

11. Etzioni, ibid., p. 24.

12. Etzioni, 1998, op. cit., p. xvi.

13. C. Lasch, *The Culture of Narcissism* (New York: W. W. Norton, 1978).

14. Etzioni, 1993, op. cit., p. 24.

15. R. Bellah et al., *Habits of the Heart: Individualism and Commitment in American Life* (Berkeley: University of California Press, 1985), p. 142.

16. See, for example, S. Pfohl, *Death at the Parasite Cafe* (New York: St.

Martin's, 1992) and S. Gottschalk, "Uncomfortably numb: Countercultural impulses in the postmodern era," *Symbolic Interaction* 16 (1993): 351–78.

17. Z. Bauman, *Mortality, Immortality, and Other Life Strategies* (Stanford, CA: Stanford University Press, 1992), p. 167.

18. Recent critiques of a national and global corporate ascendancy and its impact on the nature of work can be found in C. Derber, *Corporation Nation* (New York: St. Martin's Press, 1998) and R. Sennett, *The Corrosion of Character* (New York: W. W. Norton, 1998).

19. P. Benner and S. Gordon, "Caring practice," in S. Gordon, P. Benner, and N. Noddings (eds.), *Caregiving: Readings in Knowledge, Practice, and Politics* (Philadelphia: University of Pennsylvania Press, 1996), p. 50.

20. R. Wuthnow, *Acts of Compassion: Caring for Others and Helping Ourselves* (Princeton, NJ: Princeton University Press, 1991).

21. See P. Schervish, *Taking Giving Seriously* (Indianapolis: Indiana University Center on Philanthropy, 1993) and P. Schervish, *Care and Community in Modern Society* (San Francisco: Jossey-Bass, 1995).

22. Wuthnow, op. cit., p. 17.

23. C. Clark, *Misery and Company: Sympathy in Everyday Life* (Chicago: University of Chicago Press, 1997).

24. R. Jacoby, *Social Amnesia* (Boston: Beacon Press, 1975), quoted in L. Rubin, *Intimate Strangers: Men and Women Together* (New York: HarperCollins, 1983), p. 4.

25. The romantic love ideal, formulated in France and Germany during the twelfth century, filtered down from the nobility to the lower classes over the centuries. In its pure form the ideal of romantic love involves the notion that there is only one person in all the world we are meant to love.

26. C. Castano, "When Fairy Tales Grow Up" (Unpublished senior honor's thesis: Boston College, 1990).

27. C. W. Mills, "Situated actions and vocabularies of motive," in J. Manis and B. Meltzer (eds.), *Symbolic Interaction* (Boston: Allyn and Bacon, 1972).

28. See O. Klapp, *The Collective Search for Identity* (New York: Holt, Rinehart, and Winston, 1969).

29. M. Albom, *Tuesdays with Morrie* (New York: Doubleday, 1997).

30. It is interesting to observe that the kind of public, community death that gained Morrie such attention at the end of his life was the norm for the way people died during the Middle Ages. The social historian Phillipe Aries points out that people in the late Middle Ages and the Renaissance period actively participated in their own dying process. Dying was an open, public, and collective community process. See P. Aries, "The reversal of death: Changes in attitudes toward death in western societies," in D. Stan-

nard (ed.), *Death in America* (Philadelphia: University of Pennsylvania Press, 1975). Death has shifted from being a moral, religious, community event to a technological event. In North America, most especially, "death is a technical matter, a failure of technology in rescuing the body." See, E. Cassell, "Dying in technological society," in P. Steinfels and R. Veatch (eds.), *Death Inside Out* (New York: Harper and Row, 1975), p. 31.

31. See C. Derber, op. cit., p. 12.

32. See C. Derber, ibid., p. 12.

33. R. Sennett, *Families Against the City* (New York: Vintage Books, 1970).

34. Ibid., p. 50.

35. C. Lasch, *Haven in a Heartless World* (New York: Basic Books, 1977).

36. K. Jackson, *Crabgrass Frontier: The Suburbanization of the United States* (New York: Oxford University Press, 1985), p. 50.

37. Ibid., p. 58.

38. The terms of the debate center on whether men and women are somehow different from each other by nature or whether all behavioral differences arise from processes of socialization. One version of feminist theory argues that the only thing that distinguishes the social positions and roles of women is the lack of equality between men and women. The goal of activists holding this position is to equalize opportunities so that women might have a full range of choices. Another version of social science writing on women's roles, based in developmental psychology, argues that there are essential differences in the moral development of men and women, that men and women perceive the world in fundamentally different ways. Although writers such as Carol Gilligan stop short of arguing that differences between men and woman reflect "natural," genetic differences, this is the logical inference from their work. See C. Gilligan, *In a Different Voice: Psychological Theory and Women's Development* (Cambridge, MA: Harvard University Press, 1982). For an essay that describes these different "camps," see S. Gordon, "Feminism and caring," in S. Gordon, P. Benner, and N. Noddings (eds.), *Caregiving: Readings in Knowledge, Practice, and Politics* (Philadelphia: University of Pennsylvania Press, 1996), pp. 256–277. Another useful article on gender and caring is Rannveig Transtadottir's "Mothers who care: Gender, disability, and family life," *Journal of Family Issues*, 12 (1991): 211–28.

39. S. Gordon, 1996, op. cit., p. 273.

40. For example, W. Bennett, *The Book of Virtues: A Treasury of Great Moral Stories* (New York: Simon and Schuster, 1993).

41. J. Finch, *Family Obligations and Social Change* (Cambridge, UK: Polity Press, 1989), p. 242.

42. P. Berger and T. Luckmann, *The Social Construction of Reality* (Garden City, NY: Anchor Books, 1967).

43. See R. Shilts, *And the Band Played On: Politics, People, and the AIDS Epidemic* (New York: St. Martin's Press, 1987).

44. M. Foucault, *Madness and Civilization: A History of Insanity in the Age of Reason* (New York: Vintage Books, 1973).

45. See E. Goffman, *Asylums: Essays on the Social Situation of Mental Patients* (Garden City, NY: Doubleday Anchor, 1961); T. Szasz, *Ideology and Insanity* (Garden City, NY: Anchor Books, 1970); R. Laing, *The Politics of Experience* (New York: Ballantine Books, 1967), and T. Scheff, *Being Mentally Ill* (Chicago: Aldine, 1966).

46. See P. Conrad and J. Schneider, *Deviance and Medicalization* (St. Louis, MO: Mosby, 1980).

47. See P. Caplan, *They Say You're Crazy* (Reading, MA: Addison-Wesley, 1995).

48. R. Isaac and V. Armat, *Madness in the Streets: How Psychiatry and the Law Abandoned the Mentally Ill* (New York: Free Press, 1990), p. 250.

49. H. Lefley, *Family Caregiving in Mental Illness* (Thousand Oaks, CA: Sage Publications, 1996), pp. 186–87.

50. See, for example, B. Winick, "On autonomy: Legal and psychological perspectives," *Villanova Law Review* 37 (1992): 1705–77.

51. Lefley, op. cit.

52. See W. Ryan, *Blaming the Victim* (New York: Vintage Books, 1976).

53. For example, J. Bradshaw, *Coming Home: Reclaiming and Championing Your Inner Child* (New York: Doubleday, 1992).

54. Years ago the sociologists Talcott Parsons and Rene Fox predicted that the "nuclear family" would not be able to bear the burdens placed on it as societies modernized. See T. Parsons and R. Fox, "Illness, therapy, and the modern urban American family," *Journal of Social Issues* 8 (1952): 31–44.

55. Wolfe, op. cit., p. 54.

56. S. Hewlett and C. West, *The War Against Parents* (New York: Chapters Publications, 1998).

57. Derber, 1998, op. cit., p. 156.

58. This statement comes from Ralph Nader and was quoted in Derber, ibid., p. 156.

59. G. Simmel, "The metropolis and mental life," in K. Wolff (ed.), *The Sociology of Georg Simmel* (Glencoe, IL: The Free Press, 1950), p. 411.

60. G. Simmel, ibid., p. 410.

REFERENCES

Abel, E. and M. Nelson (eds.). 1990. *Circles of Care*. Albany: State University of New York Press.

Abosh, B. and A. Collins (eds.). 1996. *Mental Illness in the Family*. Toronto: University of Toronto Press.

Albom, M. 1997. *Tuesdays with Morrie*. New York: Doubleday.

Archer, D. and M. Constanza. 1988. *The Interpersonal Perception Task*. Berkeley: University of California Extension Media Center.

―――. 1989. "Interpreting the expressive behavior of others: The interpersonal perception task." *Journal of Nonverbal Behavior* 13: 225–45.

Aries, P. 1975. "The reversal of death: Changes in attitudes toward death in western societies." In D. Stannard (ed.), *Death in America*. Philadelphia: University of Pennsylvania Press.

Badger, T. 1996a. "Family members' experiences living with members with depression." *Western Journal of Nursing Research* 18: 149–71.

―――. 1996b. "Living with depression: Family members' experiences and treatment needs." *Journal of Psychosocial Nursing and Mental Health Research* 34: 21–29.

Baker, P., W. Yoels, J. Clair, and R. Allman. 1997. "Laughter in triadic geriatric medical encounters." In D. Franks, R. Erickson, and B. Cuthberson-Johnson (eds.), *Social Perspectives on Emotion*. Greenwich, CT: JAI Press.

Barondes, S. 1998. *Mood Genes: Hunting for the Origins of Mania and Depression*. New York: W. W. Freeman.

Bassoff, E. 1988. *Mothers and Daughters: Loving and Letting Go.* New York: Penguin Books.

Bauman, Z. 1992. *Mortality, Immortality, and Other Life Strategies.* Stanford, CA: Stanford University Press.

Beattie, M. 1992. *Codependent No More.* San Francisco: Harper San Francisco.

Becker, H., E. Hughes, and B. Geer. 1961. *Boys in White: Student Culture in Medical School.* Chicago: University of Chicago Press.

Bellah, R. et al. 1985. *Habits of the Heart: Individualism and Commitment in American Life.* Berkeley: University of California Press.

Benner, P. and S. Gordon. 1996. "Caring practice." In S. Gordon, P. Benner, and N. Noddings (eds.), *Caregiving: Readings in Knowledge, Practice, and Politics.* Philadelphia: University of Pennsylvania Press.

Bennett, W. 1993. *The Book of Virtues: A Treasury of Great Moral Stories.* New York: Simon and Schuster.

Berger, P. 1963. *Invitation to Sociology.* Garden City, NY: Doubleday.

Berger, P. and B. Berger. 1975. *Sociology: A Biographical Approach.* New York: Basic Books.

Berger, P. and T. Luckmann. 1967. *The Social Construction of Reality.* Garden City, NY: Anchor Books.

Berry, W. 1995. "Health is membership." *Utne Reader* (September–October): 60–65.

Bettelheim, B. 1979. *Surviving and Other Essays.* New York: Knopf.

Blau, P. 1955. *The Dynamics of Bureaucracy: A Study of Interpersonal Relations in Two Government Agencies.* Chicago: University of Chicago Press.

———. 1964. *Exchange and Power in Social Life.* New York: John Wiley.

Blumenthal, S. and D. Kupfer (eds.). 1990. *Suicide Over the Life Cycle: Risk Factors, Assessment, and Treatment of Suicidal Patients.* Washington, DC: American Psychiatric Press.

Blumer, H. 1969. *Symbolic Interaction: Perspective and Method.* Englewood Cliffs, NJ: Prentice-Hall.

Bogdan, R. and S. Taylor. 1987. "Toward a sociology of acceptance: The other side of the sociology of deviance." *Social Policy* (Fall): 34–39.

———. 1989. "Relationships with severely disabled people: The social construction of humanness." *Social Problems* 36 (April): 135–48.

Bottomore, T. and M. Rubel (eds.). 1956. *Karl Marx: Selected Writings in Sociology and Social Philosophy.* London: C. A. Watts.

Boynkin, A. and J. Winland-Brown. 1995. "The dark side of caring: Challenges of caregiving." *Journal of Gerontological Nursing* 21: 13–18.

Bradshaw, J. 1992. *Coming Home: Reclaiming and Championing Your Inner Child*. New York: Doubleday.

Brown, E. 1989. *My Parent's Keeper*. Oakland, CA: New Harbinger Publications.

Brown, P. 1985. *The Transfer of Care: Psychiatric Deinstitutionalization and Its Aftermath*. Boston: Routledge and Kegan Paul.

————. 1987. "Diagnostic conflict and contradiction in psychiatry." *Journal of Health and Social Behavior* 28: 37–50.

Caplan, P. 1995. *They Say You're Crazy*. Reading, MA: Addison-Wesley.

Caserta, M., D. Lund, and S. Wright. 1996. "Exploring the caregiver burden inventory (cbi): Further evidence for a multidimensional view of burden." *International Journal of Aging and Human Development* 43: 21–34.

Cassell, E. 1975. "Dying in technological society." In P. Steinfels and R. Veatch (eds.), *Death Inside Out*. New York: Harper and Row.

Castano, C. 1990. *When Fairy Tales Grow Up*. Unpublished senior honor's thesis: Boston College.

Charmaz, C. and D. Paternini (eds.). 1999. *Health, Illness, and Healing: Society, Social Context, and Self*. Los Angeles: Roxbury Publishing Company.

Christian-Smith, L. 1990. *Becoming a Woman Through Romance*. Boston: Routledge and Kegan Paul.

Clair, J., D. Karp, and W. Yoels. 1993. *Experiencing the Life Cycle: A Social Psychology of Aging*. Springfield, IL: Charles Thomas.

Clark, C. 1990. "Emotions and micropolitics in everyday life: Some patterns and paradoxes of 'place.'" In T. Kemper (ed.), *Research Agendas in the Sociology of Emotions*. Albany: State University of New York Press.

————. 1997. *Misery and Company: Sympathy in Everyday Life*. Chicago: University of Chicago Press.

Cohen, M. 1996. *Dirty Details: The Days and Nights of a Well Spouse*. Philadelphia: Temple University Press.

Collins, R. 1981. "On the microfoundations of macrosociology." *American Journal of Sociology* 86: 984–1014.

Conrad, P. (ed.). 1997. *The Sociology of Health and Illness*. New York: St. Martin's Press.

Conrad, P. and J. Schneider. 1980. *Deviance and Medicalization*. St. Louis, MO: Mosby.

Cooley, C. 1964. *Human Nature and the Social Order*. New York: Schocken.

Coyne, J., et al. 1987. "Living with a depressed person." *Journal of Consulting and Clinical Psychology* 55: 347–52.

Daniels, A. 1987. "Invisible work." *Social Problems* 34: 403–15.

Degler, C. 1991. *In Search of Human Nature*. New York: Oxford University Press.

Denzin, N. 1984. "Emotions as lived experience." *Symbolic Interaction* 8: 223–40.

———. 1989. *Interpretive Biography*. Newbury Park, CA: Sage Publications.

———. 1990. "On understanding emotion." In T. Kemper (ed.), *Research Agendas in the Sociology of Emotions*. Albany: State University of New York Press.

Derber, C. 1996. *The Wilding of America: How Greed and Violence Are Eroding Our National Character*. New York: St. Martin's Press.

———. 1998. *Corporation Nation*. New York: St. Martin's Press.

Derber, C., W. Schwartz, and Y. Magrass. 1990. *Power in the Highest Degree: Professionals and the Rise of a New Mandarin Class*. New York: Oxford University Press.

Devault, M. 1991. *Feeding the Family: The Social Organization of Caring as Gendered Work*. Chicago: University of Chicago Press.

Di Leonardo, M. 1987. "The female world of cards and holidays: Women, families and the work of kinship." *Signs* 12: 40–53.

Duff, K. 1993. *The Alchemy of Illness*. New York: Bell Tower.

Duke, P. 1992. *A Brilliant Madness: Living with Manic-Depressive Illness*. New York: Bantam Books.

Durkheim, E. 1966. *Suicide*. New York: Free Press.

Eisely, L. 1958. *Darwin's Century: Evolution and the Men Who Discovered It*. Garden City, NY: Doubleday.

Ellis, C. 1995. *Final Negotiations: A Story of Love, Loss, and Chronic Illness*. Philadelphia: Temple University Press.

Erikson, K. 1976. *Everything in Its Path*. New York: Simon and Schuster.

———. 1989. "On sociological prose." *The Yale Review* 78: 525–38.

Etzioni, A. 1993. *The Spirit of Community: The Reinvention of America Society*. New York: Simon and Schuster.

———. 1998. *The Essential Communitarian Reader*. Lanham, MD: Rowman and Littlefield Publishers.

Fadden, G., P. Bebbington, and L. Kuipers. 1987. "Caring and its burdens: A study of the spouses of depressed people." *British Journal of Psychiatry* 151: 660–67.

Finch, J. 1989. *Family Obligations and Social Change*. Cambridge, UK: Polity Press.

Finch, J. and D. Groves (eds.). 1983. *A Labour of Love: Women, Work and Caring*. London: Routledge and Kegan Paul.

Firestone, R. 1997. *Suicide and the Inner Voice: Risk Assessment, Treatment, and Case Management.* Thousand Oaks, CA: Sage Publications.

Foucault, M. 1973. *Madness and Civilization: A History of Insanity in the Age of Reason.* New York: Vintage Books.

Frank, A. 1991. *At the Will of the Body.* New York: Houghton Mifflin.

———. 1995. *The Wounded Storyteller.* Chicago: University of Chicago Press.

Frankl, V. 1988. *Man's Search for Meaning.* New York: Pocket Books.

Franks, D. 1989. "Power and role-taking." In D. Franks and D. McCarthy (eds.), *The Sociology of Emotion.* Greenwich, CT: JAI Press.

Franks, D. (series ed.). 1995. *Social Perspectives on Emotion.* Greenwich, CT: JAI Press.

Fraser, S. (ed.). 1995. *The Bell Curve Wars: Race, Intelligence, and the Future of America.* New York: Basic Books.

Freidson, E. 1970. *Profession of Medicine.* New York: Dodd, Mead.

Freud, S. 1988. *Civilization and Its Discontents.* New York: W. W. Norton.

Garfinkel, H. 1967. *Studies in Ethnomethodology.* Englewood Cliffs, NJ: Prentice-Hall.

Gergen, K. 1991. *The Saturated Self: Dilemmas of Identity in Contemporary Life.* New York: Basic Books.

Gilligan, C. 1982. *In a Different Voice: Psychological Theory and Women's Development.* Cambridge: Harvard University Press.

Gitter, G., H. Black and D. Mostofsky. 1972. "Race and sex in the communication of emotion." *Journal of Social Psychology* 88: 273–76.

Glaser, B. and A. Strauss. 1965. *Awareness of Dying.* Chicago: Aldine.

———. 1967. *The Discovery of Grounded Theory.* Chicago: Aldine.

———. 1968. *Time for Dying.* Chicago: Aldine.

Goffman, E. 1961. *Asylums: Essays on the Social Situation of Mental Patients.* Garden City, NY: Doubleday Anchor.

———. 1963. *Behavior in Public Places.* New York: Free Press.

Gordon, S. 1990. "Social structural effects on emotion." In T. Kemper (ed.), *Research Agendas in the Sociology of Emotions.* Albany: State University of New York Press.

———. 1996. "Feminism and caring." In S. Gordon, P. Benner, and N. Noddings (eds.), *Caregiving: Readings in Knowledge, Practice, and Politics.* Philadelphia: University of Pennsylvania Press.

Gordon, S., P. Benner, and N. Noddings (eds.). 1996. *Caregiving: Readings in Knowledge, Practice, and Politics.* Philadelphia: University of Pennsylvania Press.

Gottschalk, S. 1993. "Uncomfortably numb: Countercultural impulses in the postmodern era." *Symbolic Interaction* 16: 351–78.

Gramsci, A. 1980. *Selections from the Prison Notebooks*. New York: International Publishers.

Greenberg, J., et al. 1993. "Mothers caring for an adult child with schizophrenia: The effects of subjective burden on maternal health." *Family Relations* 42: 205–11.

Gubrium, J. 1991. *The Mosaic of Care: Frail Elderly and Their Families in the Real World*. New York: Springer.

Gubrium, J. and J. Holstein. 1990. *What Is Family?* Mountain View, CA: Mayfield.

Hall, R. 1991. *Organizations: Structure, Processes, and Outcomes*. Englewood Cliffs, NJ: Prentice-Hall.

Hannon, B. 1997. *Agents in My Brain: How I Survived Manic Depression*. Chicago: Open Court.

Hatfield, A. and H. Lefley (eds.). 1987. *Families of the Mentally Ill*. New York: Guilford Press.

Harré, R. and W. Parrott (eds.). 1996. *The Emotions: Social, Cultural, and Biological Dimensions*. Thousand Oaks, CA: Sage Publications.

Herrnstein, R. and C. Murray. 1994. *The Bell Curve: Intelligence and Class Structure in American Life*. New York: Free Press.

Hewitt, J. 1996. *Self and Society*. Boston: Allyn and Bacon.

Hewlett, S. and C. West. 1998. *The War Against Parents*. New York: Chapters Publications.

Hobbes, T. 1961. *Leviathan*. New York: Penguin Books. Edited by C. B. MacPherson.

Hochschild, A. 1979. "Emotion work, feeling rules, and social structure." *American Journal of Sociology* 85: 551–75.

———. 1983. *The Managed Heart: Commercialization of Human Feeling*. Berkeley: University of California Press.

———. 1990. "Ideology and emotion management: A perspective and path for future research." In T. Kemper (ed.), *Research Agendas in the Sociology of Emotions*. Albany: State University of New York Press.

Hoffman, M. 1989. "Empathic Emotions of Justice in Society." *Social Justice Research* 3(4): 283–311.

Holmstrom, L. and A. Burgess. 1978. *The Victim of Rape: Institutional Reactions*. New York: John Wiley.

Homans, G. 1961. *Human Behavior: Its Elementary Forms*. New York: Harcourt, Brace, 1961.

Isaac, R. and V. Armat. 1990. *Madness in the Streets: How Psychiatry and the Law Abandoned the Mentally Ill*. New York: Free Press.

Jackson, K. 1985. *Crabgrass Frontier: The Suburbanization of the United States*. New York: Oxford University Press.

Jacoby, R. 1975. *Social Amnesia*. Boston: Beacon Press.

Jacoby, R. and N. Glauberman (eds.). 1995. *The Bell Curve Debate: History, Documents, Opinions*. New York: Times Books.

James, V. and J. Gabe. 1996. *Health and the Sociology of Emotions*. Oxford, UK: Blackwell Publishers.

Jamison, K. 1995. *An Unquiet Mind*. New York: Knopf.

Johnson, A. 1990. *Out of Bedlam: The Truth About Deinstitutionalization*. New York: Basic Books.

Johnson, J. 1994. *Hidden Victims, Hidden Healers*. Edina, MN: Pema Publishing Co.

Kafka, F. 1998. *The Trial*. New York: Schocken Books.

Kaminer, W. 1990. "Chances are you're co-dependent too." *New York Times Book Review* (February): 1, 26ff.

Karp, D. 1973. "Hiding in pornographic bookstores: A reconsideration of the nature of urban anonymity." *Urban Life and Culture* 4: 427–51.

———. 1992. "Illness ambiguity and the search for meaning: A case study of a self-help group for affective disorders." *Journal of Contemporary Ethnography* 21: 139–70.

———. 1993. "Taking anti-depressant medications: Resistance, trial commitment, conversion, disenchantment." *Qualitative Sociology* 16: 337–59.

———. 1994. "Living with depression: Illness and identity turning points." *Qualitative Health Research* 4 (February): 6–30.

———. 1996. *Speaking of Sadness: Depression, Disconnection, and the Meanings of Illness*. New York: Oxford University Press.

Karp, D., L. Holmstrom, and P. Gray. 1998. "Leaving home for college: Expectations for selective reconstruction of self." *Symbolic Interaction* 21: 253–76.

Karp, D., G. Stone, and W. Yoels. 1991. *Being Urban: A Sociology of City Life*. New York: Praeger.

Karp D. and W. Yoels. 1976. "The college classroom: Some observations on the meanings of student participation." *Sociology and Social Research* 60 (July): 421–39.

———. 1993. *Sociology in Everyday Life*. Itasca, IL: Peacock Publishing Co.

Keitner, G. (ed.). 1990. *Depression and Families: Impact and Treatment*. Washington, DC: American Psychiatric Press.

Keitner, G., et al. 1987. "Family functioning and the course of major depression." *Comprehensive Psychiatry* 28: 54–64.

Kemper, T. 1981. "Social constructionist and positivist approaches to the sociology of emotions." *American Journal of Sociology* 87: 336–62.

Kemper, T. (ed.). 1990. *Research Agendas in the Sociology of Emotions.* Albany: State University of New York Press.

Kimmel, M. 1996. *Manhood in America: A Cultural History.* New York: The Free Press.

Kimmel, M. and M. Messner (eds.). 1989. *Men's Lives.* New York: Macmillan.

Kirk, S. and H. Kutchens. 1992. *The Selling of DSM: The Rhetoric of Science in Psychiatry.* New York: Aldine DeGreuter.

Klapp, O. 1969. *The Collective Search for Identity.* New York: Holt, Rinehart, and Winston.

Krach, P. and J. Brooks. 1995. "Identifying the responsibilities and needs of working adults who are primary caregivers." *Journal of Gerontological Nursing* 21: 41–50.

Kramer, P. 1993. *Listening to Prozac.* New York: Viking.

Krause, E. 1996. *Death of the Guilds: Professions, States, and the Advance of Capitalism.* New Haven, CT: Yale University Press.

Laing, R. 1967. *The Politics of Experience.* New York: Ballantine Books.

Lamb, W. 1998. *I Know This Much Is True.* New York: HarperCollins.

Larson, C. 1977. *Major Themes in Sociological Theory.* New York: David McKay.

Lasch, C. 1977. *Haven in a Heartless World.* New York: Basic Books.

———. 1978. *The Culture of Narcissism.* New York: W. W. Norton.

———. 1980. "Life in the therapeutic state." *New York Review of Books* (June 12): 24–31.

Lee, P., D. Soffel, and H. Luft. 1997. "Costs and coverage: Pressure toward health care reform." In P. Conrad (ed.), *The Sociology of Health and Illness.* New York: St. Martin's Press.

Lefley, H. 1996. *Family Caregiving in Mental Illness.* Thousand Oaks, CA: Sage.

Lerner, M. 1975. "The Justice Motive in Social Behavior." *Journal of Social Issues* 31(3): 1–20.

Lyman, K. 1993. *Day In, Day Out with Alzheimer's: Stress in Caregiving Relationships.* Philadelphia: Temple University Press.

Mairs, N. 1986. *Plaintext Essays.* Tucson: University of Arizona Press.

Manning, M. 1996. "Invisible wounds." *The New York Times Book Review* (January 21): 29.

Manstead, S. 1991. "Expressiveness as an individual difference." In R. Feldman and B. Rime (eds.), *Fundamentals of Nonverbal Behavior.* New York: Cambridge University Press.

Mead, G. H. 1934. *Mind, Self, and Society.* Chicago: University of Chicago Press.

Mead, M. 1961. *Coming of Age in Samoa*. New York: Morrow.

Merton, R. 1938. "Social structure and anomie." *American Sociological Review* 3: 672–82.

Merton, R. 1949. *Social Theory and Social Structure*. Glencoe, IL: The Free Press.

Miller, I., et al. 1992. "Depressed patients with dysfunctional families: Description and course of illness." *Journal of Abnormal Psychology* 101: 637–46.

Mills, C. W. 1959. *The Sociological Imagination*. New York: Oxford University Press.

———. 1972. "Situated actions and vocabularies of motive." In J. Manis and B. Meltzer (eds.), *Symbolic Interaction*. Boston: Allyn and Bacon.

Moore, T. 1992. *Care of the Soul*. New York: HarperCollins.

Neugarten, B., J. Moore, and J. Lowe. 1965. "Age norms, age constraints, and adult socialization." *American Journal of Sociology* 70: 710–17.

Neugeboren, J. 1997. *Imagining Robert: My Brother, Madness and Survival*. New York: William Morrow.

Nippert-Eng, C. 1996. *Home and Work*. Chicago: University of Chicago Press.

Nisbet, R. 1966. *The Sociological Tradition*. New York: Basic Books.

Noddings, N. 1984. *Caring: A Feminine Ethics and Moral Education*. Berkeley: University of California Press.

Noonan, A., S. Tennstedt, and F. Rebelsky. 1996. "Making the best of it: Themes of meaning among informal caregivers to the elderly." *Journal of Aging Studies* 10(4): 313–27.

O'Connor, R. 1997. *Undoing Depression*. Boston: Little, Brown.

Olesen, V. 1989. "Cargiving, ethical and informal." *Journal of Health and Social Behavior* 30: 1–10.

Papolos, D. and J. Papolos. 1992. *Overcoming Depression*. New York: HarperCollins.

Parsons, T. 1954. *Essays in Sociological Theory*. Glencoe, IL: The Free Press.

Parsons, T. and R. Fox. 1952. "Illness, therapy, and the modern urban American family." *Journal of Social Issues* 8: 31–44.

Pfohl, S. 1978. *Predicting Dangerousness: The Social Construction of Psychiatric Reality*. Lexington, MA: Lexington Books.

———. 1992. *Death at the Parasite Cafe*. New York: St. Martin's Press.

Plath, S. 1972. *The Bell Jar*. New York: Bantam.

Prus, R. 1996. *Symbolic Interaction and Ethnographic Research: Intersubjectivity and the Study of Human Lived Experience*. Albany: State University of New York Press.

Reynolds, L. 1990. *Interactionism: Exposition and Critique.* Dix Hills, NY: General Hall.

Rieff, P. 1966. *Triumph of the Therapeutic.* New York: Harper and Row.

Rosenhan, D. L. 1992. "On being sane in insane places." In C. Clark and H. Robboy (eds.), *Social Interaction.* New York: St. Martin's Press.

Rosenthal, R., et al. 1974. "Body talk and tone of voice: The language without words." *Psychology Today* 8 (September): 64–68.

Rothman, D. 1997. "A century of failure: Health care reform in America." In P. Conrad (ed.), *The Sociology of Health and Illness.* New York: St. Martin's Press.

Rubin L. 1983. *Intimate Strangers: Men and Women Together.* New York: HarperCollins.

Ryan, W. 1976. *Blaming the Victim.* New York: Vintage Books.

Scheff, T. 1966. *Being Mentally Ill.* Chicago: Aldine.

Schervish, P. 1993. *Taking Giving Seriously.* Indianapolis: Indiana University Center on Philanthropy.

———. 1995. *Care and Community in Modern Society.* San Francisco: Jossey-Bass.

Schott, S. 1979. "Emotion and social life: A symbolic interactionist analysis." *American Journal of Sociology* 84: 1317–34.

Schutz, A. 1960. *Collected Papers: Studies in Social Theory.* The Hague: Martinus Nijhoff.

Sennett, R. 1970. *Families Against the City.* New York: Vintage Books.

———. 1998. *The Corrosion of Character.* New York: W. W. Norton.

Shilts, R. 1987. *And the Band Played On: Politics, People, and the AIDS Epidemic.* New York: St. Martin's Press.

Shorter, E. 1997. *History of Psychiatry.* New York: John Wiley.

Simmel, G. 1950a. "Faithfulness and gratitude." In K. Wolff (ed.), *The Sociology of Georg Simmel.* Glencoe, IL: The Free Press.

———. 1950b. "The metropolis and mental life." In K. Wolff (ed.), *The Sociology of Georg Simmel.* Glencoe, IL: The Free Press.

———. 1950c. "The study of social forms." In K. Wolff (ed.), *The Sociology of Georg Simmel.* Glencoe, IL: The Free Press.

Simon, C. 1997. *Mad House.* New York: Random House.

Skaff, M. and L. Pearlin. 1992. "Caregivers: Role engulfment and the loss of self." *The Gerontologist* 32: 656–64.

Slater, L. 1996. *Welcome to My Country.* New York: Random House.

———. 1998. *Prozac Diary.* New York: Random House.

Smigel, E. 1969. *The Wall Street Lawyer: Professional Organization Man?* Bloomington: University of Indiana Press.

Smith, A. 1976. *Theory of Moral Sentiments*. Indianapolis, IN: Liberty Classics.

Spock, B. 1946. *The Common Sense Book of Child and Baby Care*. New York: Pocket Books.

Stommel, M., C. Given, and B. Given. 1990. "Depression as an overriding variable explaining caregiver burden." *Journal of Aging and Health* 2: 81–102.

Strauss, A. 1978. *Negotiations: Varieties, Contexts, Processes, and Social Order*. San Francisco: Jossey-Bass.

———. 1992. "Turning points in identity." In C. Clark and H. Robboy (eds.), *Social Interaction*. New York: St. Martin's.

Styron, W. 1990. *Darkness Visible: A Memoir of Madness*. New York: Random House.

Szasz, T. 1970. *Ideology and Insanity*. Garden City, NY: Anchor Books.

———. 1994. *Cruel Compassion: Psychiatric Control of Society's Unwanted*. New York: John Wiley.

Tannen, D. 1990. *You Just Don't Understand: Men and Women in Conversation*. New York: William Morrow.

Thoits, P. 1990. "Emotional deviance: Research agendas." In T. Kemper (ed.). *Research Agendas in the Sociology of Emotions*. Albany: State University of New York Press.

Thomas, D., D. Franks, and J. Calanico. 1972. "Role-taking and power in social psychology." *American Sociological Review* 37: 605–15.

Thorne, B. and Z. Luria. 1986. "Sexuality and gender in children's daily worlds." *Social Problems* 33: 176–90.

Tönnies, F. 1940. *Fundamental Concepts of Sociology*. Translated and supplemented by Charles F. Loomis. New York: American Book Company.

Torrey, E. 1997. *Out of the Shadows: Confonting America's Mental Illness Crisis*. New York: John Wiley.

Transtadottir, R. 1991. "Mothers who care: Gender, disability, and family life." *Journal of Family Issues* 12: 211–28.

Vaughan, D. 1986. *Uncoupling: Turning Points in Intimate Relationships*. New York: Oxford University Press.

———. 1996. *The Challenger Launch Decision: Risky Technology, Culture, and Deviance at NASA*. Chicago: University of Chicago Press.

Waldrop, J. 1989. "Who are the caregivers?" *American Demographics* 11: 39.

Weber, M. 1946. "Bureaucracy." In H. Gerth and C. W. Mills (eds.), *From Max Weber: Essays in Sociology*. New York: Oxford University Press.

———. 1947. *The Theory of Social and Economic Organization*. New York: Oxford University Press.

Wilson, W. 1987. *The Truly Disadvantaged: The Inner City, the Underclass, and Public Policy.* Chicago: University of Chicago Press.

Winick, B. 1992. "On autonomy: Legal and psychological perspectives." *Villanova Law Review* 37: 1705–77.

Wolfe, A. 1989. *Whose Keeper?: Social Science and Moral Obligation.* Berkeley: University of California Press.

Wolff, K. 1950. *The Sociology of Georg Simmel.* Glencoe, IL: The Free Press.

Wright, W. 1998. *Born That Way: Genes, Behavior, Personality.* New York: Knopf.

Wurtzel, E. 1994. *Prozac Nation.* Boston: Houghton Mifflin.

Wuthnow, R. 1991. *Acts of Compassion: Caring for Others and Helping Ourselves.* Princeton, NJ: Princeton University Press.

Yoels, W. and J. Clair. 1994. "Never enough time: How medical residents manage a scarce resource." *Journal of Contemporary Ethnography* 23: 185–213.

Young, R. and E. Kahana. 1989. "Specifying caregiver outcomes: Gender and relationship aspects of caregiver strain." *The Gerontologist* 29: 660–66.

Zarit, S., P. Todd, and J. Zarit. 1986. "The subjective burden of husbands and wives as caregivers: A longitudinal study." *The Gerontologist* 26: 260–66.

Index